# Knocked Up Knocked Down

## Postcards of Miscarriage and Other Misadventures
## from the Brink of Parenthood

### by Monica Murphy LeMoine

**Published by Catalyst Book Press**
**Livermore, California**

Copyright © 2010 by Monica Murphy LeMoine
Cover Design: Kathy McInnis

Summary:  After Monica Murphy LeMoine experiences a miscarriage, she has to figure out a way to get on with her life, but finds the typical miscarriage grief literature sappy and unhelpful. LeMoine embarks on her own adventure to find healing.

Monica Muphy LeMoine has changed some names in order to protect people's privacy. Everything else is true to the best of her knowledge.

Catalyst Book Press would like to thank Corbin Lewars, Kathy McInnis, and Dennis Powers. Monica's drawings came  to us inscribed within the pages of a cookbook. We tried some of the recipes. The cinnamon rolls were particularly delicious.

ISBN 978-0-9802081-3-9
Library of Congress Control Number:  2010921280
June 2010
Printed in the United States of America

To order additional copies of the book, contact Catalyst Book Press
www.catalystbookpress.com
info@catalystbookpress.com
925-606-5992

FOR KEVIN

# The First Journey Segment:
## From a Rural Abyss of Death, Paranoia, and Loud-Ass Motorcycles
*July to December, 2006*

## Panty Focus

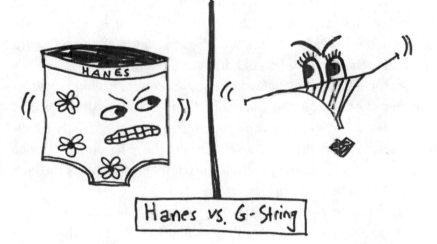

Hanes vs. G-String

TOMORROW IS A BIG DAY.

It's my first public appearance since a forceful stream of vomit traveled from my mouth into the shrubbery; an inanimate object and its bloody accoutrements flew out of my vagina; and all sorts of other waste products projected themselves loudly from my rear end into the toilet. Tomorrow, I'll return to the leafy University of Arkansas campus where Kevin and I teach English, breezily say hello to my officemates, and stand up before a classroom full of bored-looking Middle Eastern students as though nothing out of the ordinary just happened.

Only Kevin, my reasonable and soft-spoken husband of nearly four years, will know the poopy, barfy, bloody truth of the last forty-eight hours, for he was a firsthand witness of this visual-audio spectacle of mass bodily exodus. *So much for our sex life*, I recall thinking fleetingly as it was happening, comforted only by the knowledge that our early courtship involved his chivalrous rescue of me, piss-drunk and covered in human shit, from an Uzbek pit toilet. Relationship-wise, there wasn't anywhere else to go but up. And now, once again: nowhere else to go but up.

All I have to do is find the perfect pair of underwear.

It's a serious task, the choosing of the underwear. Isn't a woman's choice of underwear, after all, one of the best indicators of her own sense of aliveness? That is, her vision of herself as a tingly animate being; her confidence in her own vitality-flushed body as something worth drawing attention to; her belief in the likelihood of getting laid? With that buzzy, back-to-school feeling of nervous excitement, I've spent the last half-hour emptying every dresser drawer onto the dusty hardwood floor of our bedroom, digging through wadded up clothing in search of the pair. I know exactly which one I'm looking for.

At first glance of my undergarment choices, one would think I'm about as sexually alive as an Amish grandmother. Most of what I own is of the faded, stretched-out bloomer variety; you know, the Hanes cotton briefs that come in a plastic pouch at Target, rising up to the waist and mercifully swallowing up those love handles and paunch belly. Not the sort of underwear one would use to embellish a hot body or elicit passionate foreplay.

But somewhere among the drab Hanes, there is exactly one non-granny item that Kevin gave me this past Christmas while we were staying at my parents' house. It was a flimsy pink and red g-string—the first and only I've ever owned. I remember holding the little thong panties up to the light after opening the shiny silver package, examining their girlyness, their minimalism, and whispering, "Wow." How remarkable that my husband of nearly four years might still see me as a feminine

6

woman with a body worth sliding into a teensy-weensy thong! Me, in skimpy underwear: it wasn't a way that I had ever dared to perceive myself.

Those are precisely the panties I am hoping to wear to work tomorrow, in a bold expression of feminine hope and defiance: *vaginal expulsion or none, vomit or no vomit, excrement or no excrement: I am sexy hellcat! Hear me roar!*

But I can't seem to find them, and—as I paw through my wrinkled Hanes bloomers—my spirits begin to fall. It's late—eight o'clock already—and I'm tired. Kevin agreed to watch *Shaun of the Dead* with me tonight, even though we've seen it about ten times, so we'd better start that before we both fall asleep. Come to think of it, with my still-sore crotch and belly, I'm now feeling about as sexually charged as a dead leaf blowing around a suburban driveway. I have no business wearing thong panties at a time like this. Even the word "panties" grosses me out. Blegh.

So I give up the search for that magical and life-giving g-string, settling on pink-flowered Hanes high-risers instead. Probably best to go with the safe and conservative option for now, for the sake of practicality. There will be plenty of time to look for those Christmas panties again when my body feels back to normal.

Like I said, there ain't a damn place to go but up.

## BACK TO NORMAL

KEVIN AND I SET OUT ON THE HILLY, forty-five minute walk to the school, arriving with sweat patches on our shirts as we always do. I stop in the first-floor bathroom to hold my armpits above the blasting air conditioner and adjust my Texas-sized undies so they aren't bunched up at the top.

My three officemates are busy thumbing through textbooks and writing things down in notebooks when I step into my office. The familiar scene of teachers frantically prepping for class at the last minute: I recognize it immediately, because I'm usually a part of it. Now I feel like a ghost drifting in, an outsider returning from a long vacation to some exotic country. Everybody looks up and says "hey" in unison. I smile and toss my backpack casually onto the floor.

There's a single greeting card on my desk, open and propped up, signed by all of the teachers. On the front is a reprinted watercolor painting of a daisy. A bright, stinging line of disappointment, loneliness, zigzags through me without warning. What was I expecting? That my entire desk and chair be buried under a mountain of flowers and gifts and balloons? I feel childish in my disappointment, almost embarrassed. My mom would tell me to be a good sport. With a piece of scotch tape, I affix the card to the edge of my bookshelf so that the daisies are displayed.

"So glad you're back, Monica," says Jackie. "Gosh, you look thin!"

"Yeah," I say, proudly not missing a beat. "It's called the three-day hospital starvation diet. That'd be an awesome commercial! Somebody should patent that."

Ha, ha, ha. We all laugh. I can tell that everyone feels more at ease now that I've proven myself capable of not just holding myself together, but making a wisecrack. The relief emanating from Don and Henry is especially palpable; men are always the ones who need the most reassurance that a woman hasn't transformed into a raging emotional monster. Glad I could provide that reassurance. Taking a deep breath and exhaling, I tuck the disappointment of moments ago into the back of my mind.

The day goes by just like any other normal day, which is what I wanted, I guess. The usual chipper hellos in the hallway, the jostling of Lean Cuisine meals in the freezer to make room for my own, the sound of pleasant chit-chat trailing from the copy room. My students behave like their usual selves, sighing audibly when asked to open their grammar books, chuckling at the sight of chalk on my face. Between classes I catch fleeting glimpses of Kevin, striding around corners in his khaki pants and collared shirt with books and papers clutched under one arm.

"So, you survived," he says on our afternoon walk home, which is always sweatier than the morning commute.

"Yeah," I say. "Nobody...like...even mentioned it. Probably a good thing." There's a long period of silence as I train my eyes downward onto the glaring white sidewalk. Horizontal lines separating concrete panels go by, one after the other, and I'm averaging about two steps between each line. God, this place is hot. The warm air is heavy, and a very slight breeze rustles through the dense tree leaves above us.

Something begins to unravel inside my stomach, releasing a feeling I can't quite identify, reminiscent of how I used to feel sometimes at summer camp. Loneliness? Homesickness? I swallow, hard, suppressing a deep, unexpected sob. Today was supposed to go upward, not down.

"Mon, it's not because they don't care." Kevin inches closer to me as we wait to cross Dixon Street.

"I know," I say. "They gave me a nice card. I taped it to the bookshelf."

We hardly ever hold hands, but he takes mine now. "Don't forget, we just moved here. It's not like they know you that well."

Logically he's right, I know. But still. My lower lip trembles. "I just wish we had some real friends in this town."

"We will. These things take time. It always does when we move to a new place—you know that. It'll happen." He suddenly pulls his hand away and crouches down to adjust the strap of his sandal. "Fucking Chacos. Always digging into the same exact spot on my left toe. Every damned time."

A smile surfaces and tugs up the corners of my mouth as I watch him. It's a strange relief to know that life's usual little constants—like my husband cussing out shoes that he paid a lot of money for—still happen, keeping me anchored to something recognizable. I'm feeling strangely off-balance today, and I'll take whatever footholds of normalcy I can get.

# LOOMING THREAT OF PERSONAL EXTINCTION

GOOGLING "BRAIN CANCER SYMPTOMS" is never a good idea, but I decide to do it anyway. It's a hot and sticky late afternoon, and I'm sitting at the computer in my underwear and a t-shirt, blinds drawn to block out the glaring Arkansas sun. I can hear Kevin in the kitchen chopping vegetables, the thud of the knife coming down. It doesn't take me long to discover a list of warning signs: double vision. Headaches. Tingling or numbness in the arm. Forgetfulness. Sagging on one side of the face.

As I study this list, it becomes frighteningly apparent that I seem to be exhibiting not just one but *several* of these exact symptoms. I *have* been rather spacey lately, now that I think about it. I extend both arms and wiggle my fingers, fanning them in and out. They feel strangely numb. I get up and stand in front of the dresser mirror to examine my own face, shoulder-length hair pulled back with a rubber band, and can't help but notice that I look...different. A little bit puffier than usual, one might say saggy even, especially on the left side of my face. And I begin to notice a bit of pressure inside of my head. Nothing acutely painful; just a warm, distinct presence of something. Quite possibly, even plausibly, a brain tumor, burgeoning on the left-hand side, next to my ear.

A small seed of worry begins to form in my mind, but—like a reasonable person—I decide to do more research before jumping to conclusions. Tapping into the vast quantities of legitimate medical information available on the Internet, I discover photographs and blogs of people—even youngish, healthy-looking people like myself—who at some point discovered they had brain cancer. Some are surviving, mostly the ones who caught it early, but many are now either dead or dying. All

I can think about is that I could be one of those dead or dying if I don't act fast.

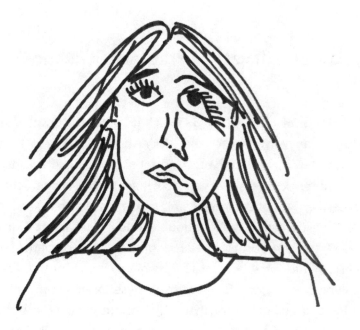

The last thing I want is to come across as a foolish, over-reactive hypochondriac, something nobody wants to be. So I express my concerns to Kevin with measured caution.

"I think something's wrong with me, Kev," I say during our walk home from work.

"What do you mean?"

"Well, I mean, I haven't been able to concentrate lately. Like, I'll get up there in front of my students and just, sort of, forget what I'm supposed to teach that day, or forget how to explain a grammar rule. Or like, the other day I was sitting in the copy room and Don came up and said something to me, and I totally lost track of the conversation—like my mind went blank."

"You *just had* a miscarriage. I think it's probably normal to feel weird."

"No, but it's really not a normal feeling. I mean, I'm over the whole miscarriage thing, so it wouldn't make sense for this to be related to that. I've also got a tingling feeling in my arm, and my face looks weird to me, and I feel something in my head."

"Something in your head?"

"Yeah, like this thing next to my ear, inside my brain. It feels like a tumor."

"You don't have a tumor, Mon."

"Yeah but…shit. I forgot what I was going to say. See? That's what I'm saying—I feel really forgetful. Like, *abnormally* forgetful."

"You don't have a tumor. What're we making for dinner tonight, by the way?"

I DECIDE TO CALL THE CONSULTING NURSE and explain my symptoms in a calm and casual way, without giving any indication that I seriously think I might be dying. My hope is that whichever doctor gets assigned my case will connect the dots on his or her own, making what I know to be the correct diagnosis—brain cancer—and call back recommending immediate surgical tumor removal.

*07-17-2006. Patient called stating her left arm and hand has a numb and tingling sensation, that the episodes come and go and have been noticeable from pregnancy loss 7/6/06. She states she is a teacher, now has difficulty concentrating, episodes of forgetfulness, anxiety episodes, feeling anxious about becoming mentally ill and feels spacey. Dr. P will call patient back with response.*

I do get a return phone call, that very same day in fact, but the diagnosis and treatment are not at all what I expect:

*07-17-2006. Lexapro 10mg #30, prescribed by Dr. P for anxiety. Patient advised to pick up Lexapro samples tomorrow and take 1 daily, with instructions to call after 2-3 weeks to report on progress.*

Lexapro? Fucking anti-anxiety meds? Since when is being assertive about one's own personal health a sign of a mental disorder? Yes, I'm anxious. But it's because I probably have brain cancer, for God's sake! Wouldn't anyone be a little anxious? I feel insulted, really.

*7-18-06. Patient has not called back, nor picked up Lexapro sample as yet.*

Damn straight I haven't picked it up, and I'm not going to. They can keep their psychiatric drug samples, thanks. With a rising feeling of determination to survive, I look up "neurologist" in the phone book. There aren't many to choose from out here in the boondocks. I dial the first number listed, not knowing or caring if I'm out of my insurance coverage network. Screw it. Somebody needs to scan my brain ASAP, and if that means dropping a little extra cash, so be it.

"Dr. Williams' office. Can I help you?"

"Yes, hi. My name is Monica LeMoine, and I'd like to schedule an MRI brain scan?"

"And who referred you?"

"Um, nobody. I mean, I didn't get a doctor's referral. But I know I need to have my brain scanned, because I'm showing symptoms of brain cancer."

Long pause. "I'm sorry, but we only work with referrals, so you'll need to get that from your doctor."

I hang up, dejected. Another roadblock. I'm starting to really feel like I'm in a death trap now. I dial the university health clinic. It's time for a fresh start with a new doctor, someone who doesn't know me at all.

"Yes, hello. I'm an instructor over at the Language Center, and I need an appointment as soon as possible. Today, if you've got something. Any doctor is fine."

"Is this a medical emergency, ma'am?"

"No—I mean, sort of, yes. I need a referral for an MRI right away."

"An MRI referral? Uh, first available is tomorrow afternoon. Will that—"

"Yes, that's fine."

After classes the next day, I find myself sitting across from a bearded man in a flowered Hawaiian shirt, his dark and stringy hair pulled back in a ponytail that hangs down to the middle of his back. The only evidence that this man is a real doctor is the stethoscope around his neck and the nametag on his shirt. He peers at me through his thick glasses.

"So, the nurse tells me you want…an MRI referral?"

"Yes."

"Because you think you might have brain cancer?"

"Yes."

"And your form here says you had…let's see….a miscarriage at almost four months gestation? That was less than two weeks ago."

"Yes."

"Four months. That's pretty far along."

"Yes."

"Looks like you…delivered the fetus vaginally?"

For the record, I hate the word 'vaginal' and all forms of it—and wish he hadn't said it. What does any of this matter anyway? How else might one deliver a fetus? "Uh-huh."

"Planned pregnancy?"

"Kinda. I mean, it would've been nice if it had worked out. Wasn't like do-or-die, though."

He has me stand up and balance on one leg, look into a bright light while he examines my pupils, and read some letters on the far wall with one eye covered up.

"I really don't see anything wrong with you, Monica. Anytime you go through something traumatic like a miscarriage, your mind can do some strange things. You've got to give your brain and body time to heal, you know."

"I know. But…" I try to hold back tears. Everything, everyone, is plotting against me, it seems. "It would really help me heal faster if, you know, you would just sign me off to get the MRI scan. Just so I could at least rule a tumor *out*. I just need some evidence, and I'll be fine."

He looks at me for a long time. "Well, I suppose I can sign the form for you, but I really recommend you wait a few weeks before you go through with this."

"Great, thanks so much," I say, instantly flooded with relief. I wipe my nose on the back of my arm and the doctor hands me a Kleenex. My plan is to make the appointment as soon as I get home, of course, for the longer I wait, the more time the tumor has to extend its ugly, deadly tentacles even farther into the reaches of my brain. The doctor's referral slip, that coveted ticket to my survival, is gingerly folded and tucked into my back pocket. I vow not to lose it.

But I'm somehow too busy to call that day, and the day after that. Things just come up: a get-together at the Crown Pub with some other teachers, a visit with my parents (who know nothing about the whole brain tumor incident, and don't need to), a trip to Eureka Springs. All of this takes my focus away from the tingling arm and sagging face and forgetfulness, and by the end of the following weekend, I've more or less forgotten about my symptoms all together.

Sunday evening, Kevin and I are rifling through a disheveled heap of papers, mostly junk mail and crumpled receipts that have been accumulating on top of the dresser, and we make two piles: "save" and "pitch." I come across that dog-eared MRI referral slip somewhere in the middle of that heap, and toss it into the "pitch" pile without a second thought. If the cancer comes back, I'm sure I can go back in to see that guy with long hair for a new referral. He seems to be on my side.

# Fetus With Fins

THERE'S A FISH POND ON THE SIDE of our little yellow house—just a five-foot hole in the ground that somebody lined with cement and painted aqua blue, filled with water, and stocked with about twenty abnormally fat, bulbous-looking goldfish with flowy tails. They were here when we arrived, thriving on their own, subsisting, I guess, on algae or bugs or whatever other edible particles might be floating around in there. I've never really taken much notice of them, other than occasionally remarking on how fascinating it is to have a self-sustaining little ecosystem in the yard.

On a scorching hot Saturday, I look out the bedroom window and notice that the water has gotten lower than ever before, and that two fish are floating belly up. I wouldn't say I feel exactly sad about their demise, but mildly disturbed and perplexed nonetheless. Kevin scoops out the dead fish and tosses them into the shrubbery in the back corner of the yard, and we begin adding water to the pond with a garden hose every other day, just to keep the water level up. Still, we keep discovering freshly deceased fish, one every couple of days. Each time we find one, Kevin adds it to the now-stinky fish graveyard in the shrubs, and I become more perturbed.

This is now an official problem for me. It's become my personal crusade to save these fluttery orange creatures with blank expressions. They are, after all, a part of our household. I begin to wonder if the problem is lack of food, and not water level. We're about to go on a three-day excursion with students to a little town called Mountain View, and I'll be damned if I allow these fish to starve while we're away.

I notice that above the water line of the pond, moving in wavy lines along the aqua blue concrete, there are little black ants—lots and lots of them. Hundreds, maybe thousands of them. Using the hose, I spray-wash the majority of them into the pond, where they form a patchy floating ant-carpet and cling to leaf fragments for their dear lives. I sort of feel sorry for those ants; what an awful predicament to be in. I wonder briefly if I'm a bad person for taking the liberty of feeding them to someone else, but when the fish gobble them up frenetically, I feel as though I've redeemed myself. Now, the fish are presumably full and happy, and the ants have been saved from a prolonged, drowning death.

Just before we board the field trip bus, I check online and discover that you're apparently not *supposed* to give fish so much food at once, because they overeat. I suppose I could have looked this up beforehand, but hindsight is always twenty-twenty, isn't it? It's not clear to me exactly what happens if they overeat. Do they explode? Become obese? Are they susceptible to adult-onset diabetes? Anyway, it's too late now.

"Kevin," I say on the bus. "I think I might have just killed the fish. I just read that you're not supposed to overfeed them."

"I think they'll be fine."

"Yeah, but what if they're all dead when we get home?"

"So what? They're fish."

He's right. Why should I care anyway? What have those fish ever done for me? I don't even *like* fish that much. Still, throughout the weekend I alternate between feeling melancholy about our lost fetus, and worried about those fish.

When we arrive home, first things first: I ask Kevin to run out and check the pond, because I'm afraid to look. He says he will after he pees, but that's much too long to wait, so I decide to brave it and check the damn thing myself. I'm sure the fish will be fine, flitting and fluttering around as usual, perhaps with one or two deceased ones floating off to the side. But that's nothing new.

I go out the back screen door and walk over to the pond's edge. Halfway there, I see it: the fish, what appears to be every single one of them, floating lifelessly on the surface of the water, their white bellies glinting in the sun. I cover my mouth and nose with my hands and breathe in sharply, feeling my stomach drop, and tiptoe over to get a closer look. Nothing is moving in that pond; it's just an island of dead, still fish.

I run inside and throw myself on the bed, sobbing quietly, feeling awful. Sad about the state of the world, the death that seems to be all around me, the profound loss of not just my fetus, but an entire clan of innocent goldfish. They were doing just fine before I started disrupting their ecosystem. I acted blindly and stupidly, without thinking about the consequences, and now we're all alone in this yellow house without any fish to keep us company. Okay, so they weren't exactly bursting with personality, but nobody deserves to get decimated. Kevin flushes the toilet and comes into the bedroom.

"They're all dead," I say into my pillow.

"All of them?"

"Yeah. I killed them. I'm a bad person."

Kevin puts his arm around me. The sane and down-to-earth me with a sense of humor, the one hiding underneath this blanket of irrational emotion, knows that her husband is trying not to smile. Normally, this is the kind of thing we'd smile about together. *Oh well*, we would say. *Darwin's law.* But he's going along with it for a while, indulging me in what he trusts is just temporary absurdity, in part because he finds it amusing, and in part because he wants me to be okay. And if this is what I need to be okay, so be it.

"No, you're not a bad person. Don't be ridiculous. Who knows why they died?"

I don't argue about it, but I know the truth. I'm a serial goldfish killer, a bad fish mommy.

Kevin goes outside and dutifully cleans up the mess of death. I can hear the bushes rustle as they are pelted with flying fish corpses. After a while, he comes back inside, leans against the doorframe and looks at me.

"There's one fish still alive," he says. "Looks pretty active."

19

I stop sniffling. "Really?"

"Uh-huh. Maybe we can buy some more fish at the pet store tomorrow to keep him company."

*One fish alive.*

This is far more serious and important than Kevin knows, for it's another opportunity to nurture someone in need, and give him a good life. A shot at salvation, at *motherhood*. I jump up and run outside to take a look at him, wiping tears off my face. Sure enough, he's in there, zipping around healthily, looking up at me. He seems smaller than the others were; perhaps he's the equivalent of a teenager in fish-years. It occurs to me briefly that this one could very well be my fetus, reincarnated in the form of a swamp creature with fins.

"I'll take care of you," I whisper, watching him move through the water in big figure-eights beneath the blue and green reflection of the trees and sky above. Kevin comes up behind me and puts his hand on my shoulder, and I feel suddenly like we're a real, living, Norman-Rockwell- style family: two parents and a fish-child.

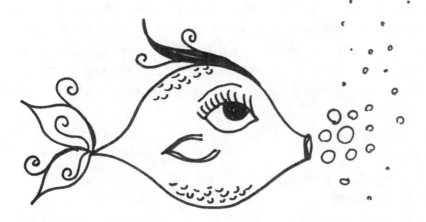

# BEER GOGGLES

OUR LITTLE FISH-CHILD LIVES FOR ALL OF twelve hours before turning belly-up like the rest.

Fucker.

Kevin doesn't seem all that upset about this fact, not that I would expect him to be. Truth be told, I don't feel much of anything either, which goes to show that my entire love affair with the goldfish clan was probably something I made up in my head. While I can't claim to understand how my mind is working these days, I do know that Arkansas is beginning to feel like a hopeless pit of death. Even the picturesque town Fayetteville oftentimes feels about as vibrant as the setting of *Children of the Corn*, mysteriously unpopulated, as though knife-wielding youngsters emerged from the surrounding countryside and obliterated everybody in sight.

Desperately seeking humanity, Kevin and I walk up the hill to Tiny Tim's, a pizza joint on the edge of the eerily quiet town square. As usual on a weeknight, the place is nearly empty. We sit at a dimly lit corner booth and lean into each other over a pitcher of amber beer, talking in low voices about normal life-related things—future plans, friends, family—and avoid the unsavory topic of dead fish. Kevin's parents have invited us to Hilton Head for Christmas, and we discuss if that's something we ought to do. They live in San Diego—his retired military dad who now does war planning as a contractor, his bubbly schoolteacher mother. I haven't talked with them personally about our recent misfortunes, not because they aren't perfectly nice people, but because I find it easier to let Kevin field those calls.

A warm and buzzy feeling courses down my neck and shoulders as I gulp down my second pint, and I feel an unexpected surge of aliveness and hope. The lights around me seem more sparkly, the waitress's smile suddenly warmer. Ahhhh, the beauty of life through beer goggles!

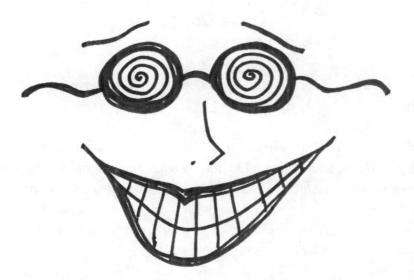

As we talk, it dawns on me: perhaps it's time to shed my tired fears and anxieties of the past month and throw a party. Not just any old party, but a huge dance party with loads of booze and thumping house music. Time to stop waiting for something better to come around, and start living!

"We don't have plans on Saturday, do we?" I ask.

"Not that I know of. Netflix."

"Good—let's have a dance party, in celebration of our five-or-whatever-week miscarriage survival mark!"

"Do we even know enough people to invite?"

Good point; we really don't have enough friends for a party bona fide party—but that doesn't seem like an insurmountable obstacle.

"Not really," I say, downing the rest of my beer and belching loudly, glancing around to see if anybody heard. No one did, of course, because we're the only customers here. "I'll just invite all the teachers. *Somebody*'ll show."

"Who's going to clean up afterward?"

"I know, I know. I will."

When we get home, I type an e-mail message to the whole faculty at our school: *You are invited to our Annual End-of-Summer Dance Party! This Saturday, 8:30pm - ? BYOB—Jello shots will be provided!*

Okay, so it isn't exactly an "annual" thing. But every annual event has to have a first time, right? I ponder for a moment if we have any other friends outside of the school—even mere acquaintances or friends of acquaintances—to add to the invite list. Nope, can't think of any. I read it over one last time, and hit "send."

THERE ARE EXACTLY SIX PEOPLE at the party, including Kevin and me. A thin crowd for our large-ish house that still doesn't have much furniture, but I've slurped down enough Jello-shots not to notice. Hip hop music blares from little speakers attached to our computer and candles flicker on the window sill, casting wavy rings of light on the wood floors. Three of us dance in the middle of the dining room, while the others cluster around the kitchen island, sipping beer and munching Fritos that I've poured into a big plastic bowl. My head spins and I close my eyes, drunk and jubilant, pretending to be the hottest dancer on stage at the biggest, booming-est club in New York City. This is how life is supposed to be, how it always was. Normal, non-dying, non-objects-flying-out-of-vagina life.

After everyone has gone, Kevin and I crawl into bed without bothering to clean up, and I burrow my face into his armpit.

"That was fun for such a small crowd," I say, hearing my own words slur together.

"Yeah. It was."

"Everyone who showed up is cool. Let's be sure we make them our friends, okay?"

"Arright. I think we can do that."

We lay there in silence, and soon I hear Kevin breathing rhythmically, already asleep and leaving me alone in my drunken mental universe. I wish he were awake, or that I were asleep with him. A flash of car lights moves across the dark ceiling, and I hear the loud screech of tires outside the house, young male voices yelling something indecipherable. Fayetteville always seems that way: quiet for the most part, with random spurts of obnoxious sound every now and then. It occurs to me how little I really know about this place.

My mood slips rather suddenly from the dance-party high of minutes ago, and I snuggle closer up against my sleeping husband. *I'm changing*, I think, *morphing into one of those moody types*. I thought I could only go upward after two days of barfing and shitting, of dazed bawling in bed, of taut phone conversations with faraway friends and family. But now I seem to only be in a worse state, worrying constantly about things not worth worrying about. Or worse, things that don't really exist.

My thoughts wander backward in time, flipping through images of the past five weeks like a cartoon booklet, freezing on a haunting picture of myself. Me in a pool of blood, eyes shiny and wide open like a wild animal trapped in a cage, hair up in a sloppy, half-assed ponytail. Kevin is hovering above me, a protective shadow.

*I don't want to see it, but can you describe it?* I see my own lips moving.

A doctor with reflective glasses, looking down between my legs, holding her fingers five inches apart as a thick cable of dark hair falls into her face.

*It looks like a baby, a miniature one,* she says matter-of-factly. *About this size.*

The scene stops there, and replays again. *A miniature one. About this size.* Stop, replay. *A miniature one. About this size.* Stop, replay.

Tears stream unstoppably out of my eyes, running down my face into the crevice where my cheek is pressed against Kevin's skin until he wakes up as he always does. Within moments I drift fretfully to sleep, and dream of that genderless, faceless mini-child rising up and out of my stomach and shooting into nighttime sky, floating away until it resembles a lonely speck in outer space. I reach for it, frantically trying to capture it in my hand so I can coddle and protect it the way a parent should, but coming up empty. That dream morphs into a loud, dark nightmare, filled with rotting fish corpses floating in the bathtub, and cancer-stricken people with pale faces and bald heads, all shouting menacingly that they're coming to get me.

At the first sign of blue morning light, I awake with an unsettled stomach, swollen eyes, and a pulsating headache. Kevin is sleeping with his arm thrown over his face. I stumble into the kitchen and start a pot of coffee, spilling grounds all over the counter top as I mutter, "Fuck," and take two extra-strength Tylenol with a glass of Alka-Seltzer—a medical double whammy. After finding a slightly soft and wilted cucumber in the back of the refrigerator, I cut two circular slices out of the middle, lie down on the living room sofa, and press the slices against my eyes.

Thank God it's not a weekday, so I can hole up and nurse myself back to a state of normalcy. Like I said before, sadness isn't going to get me anywhere. And neither will my face when it looks like that of a puffed up sea monster.

# Elusive Fineness

PEOPLE OFTEN ASK ME how Kevin is doing, hoping I have some insiders' information to which only a wife has special access. It's a fair question. I suppose I do get more physical Kevin-exposure than most people, more one-on-one time, so I ought to know something. I watch him doing ordinary things—peeling carrots for his lunch, shouting out profanity during college football, folding his shirts into perfect rectangles—and wonder if everything is okay.

Whenever I ask him how he is, he says, "Fine," and when I try to press for more information, he invariably says something like, "What do you want me to say?"

So I'm left to assume that he is, in fact, fine—and that's what I tell people who ask.

I've always wanted there to be more female emotional complexity going on inside of him than there really is. It started a long time ago, when I was resting my head on his bare chest after a bout of sex in a friend's apartment in Uzbekistan. Kevin was silently gazing at the ceiling and stroking my hair, as men sometimes do after sex. I asked him everyone's favorite girly question—"what are you thinking about?"—waiting and hoping for something like: "how I've never loved anyone more than you," or "how your hair feels like corn silk beneath my fingers." But instead, he said: "I'm trying to remember the bus schedule to Tashkent."

A disappointingly un-complicated, un-romantic response. To me, that's the equivalent of saying "fine." Just sort of a let-down, that's all.

For now, I can accept that he really is doing peachy keen (well, as peachy keen as one can be, given the circumstances), and that he is no

26

longer striving for fineness like I am, groping for a desirable mental state. I'm happy for him in a begrudging sort of way, I guess. I wish him well, way up there in that elusive land of fineness, even though he's technically a bit of an asshole for leaving me back here to fend off insanity by myself.

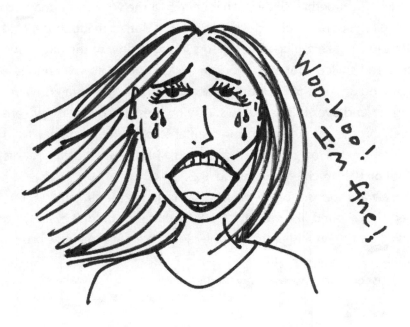

AS FOR ME, NOTHING FOLLOWS ANY sort of predictable pattern; I think I'm back to normal, and then realize I'm not. For example, when a solo trip to the grocery store ends dramatically with the inexplicable urge to cry in the canned food aisle, a dangerously fast drive home with a film of tears obscuring my vision, and an emotional meltdown in bed upon arrival, I know I'm not really fine just yet. Kevin is always there at the exact right time, draping his arm around me. Increasingly, he sounds worried at moments like these, because this is unchartered territory that neither of us quite understands. Getting randomly upset isn't something we *do* in this relationship.

Not until now, at least.

"Have you been doing this…*often*?" he asks into my hair. "Feeling this way, I mean? Running off and crying like this? All by yourself?"

"Um…" In such conversations, I get the urge to temper my response, using just the right words to reassure him that I'm not clinically depressed or anything like that. There must be only so much he can tolerate, so many times I can burst into patternless tears before he gives up and falls out of love, wondering whatever happened to the Monica he married. *That* Monica kept her cool under pressure. *That* Monica made sense. *That* Monica didn't wake me up at odd hours in the middle of the night. She laughed and smiled a lot. *That* Monica wouldn't break down crying just from picking up a can of Del Monte pineapples. *That* Monica ran forward, getting up and over things like this. I try my best to sound like we are relatively on the same page in the mental-stability department. "No, I don't feel like this too often. Just once in a while. Hey, let's drink beers barefoot on the porch—we're in Arkansas."

He always seems subtly relieved when I change the subject like that, pleased that I sound like myself again. Not that he wouldn't *mind* lying in bed all afternoon and emoting (or letting me emote to him, since he really doesn't emote like I do).

He just couldn't live that way forever.

# Brief History of a Fetus

LATELY, I'VE BEEN HAVING TROUBLE PROCESSING what a fetus actually *is*. I mean, I get what it is in a biological sense: a vaguely tadpole-like creature with an oversized head and twiggy little limbs. Simple. But there must be more to a fetus than that, because otherwise its demise wouldn't wreak so much havoc inside my head. Who cares if there's one less vaguely tadpole-like creature in the world?

For me, the best way to understand a fetus is to know that specific developing infant's history, the perfect storm of feelings and circumstances that caused egg and sperm to find each other in the first place. So I find myself staring often into space and stringing memories together, hoping they'll form a coherent image of a something—a little human being, perhaps—worth missing.

1999: I was single, aged twenty-three, and living in a tiny, dusty village in Uzbekistan with ten sheep, a handful of chickens, and a cackling old babushka who gummed her rice into swallow-able form. I was there for my two-and-a-half years of Peace Corps "service," although I didn't quite know—or care, for that matter—how teaching local school kids to say "arm" and "pen" in English actually served anyone at all. I did know that I felt tremendously content with life as it was, free of the pressures of the modern world. There were three things that occupied the bulk of my brain space: which of my two rumpled skirts to wear to school, how to avoid chomping down on pebbles that might be lurking in my rice, and how to snag Kevin LeMoine.

Kevin was a fellow volunteer. The minute I saw him climb aboard the bus that would take us all to Dulles International Airport, I knew he was the one I wanted: not to be cliché, but tall, dark and handsome—and a nice person to boot. The more I got to know him, cautiously approaching him with awkward small talk, the more I pined for him. Here was a person who wasn't afraid to go days without showering and drink to the point of barfing, yet had good social skills and at least one or two goals in life. Coincidentally, we wound up working together at an English summer camp in the dusty countryside. There, he finally figured out what I'd known all along: that we were supposed to be together, starting with a covert make-out session in the supply closet. He was the best kisser in the Central Asian steppe, from what I could tell.

We started dating. Our blissful "dates" consisted of meeting every six weeks in the capital city of Tashkent, drinking lots of beer, and gorging ourselves on roasted chicken with grease running down our arms. We would talk and belly laugh incessantly, collapsing into bed at our favorite roach-infested, dollar-a-night hotel. Whimsical, unabashed love—and lots and lots of loud sex, of course. In between these dreamlike weekends, I spent my time facing the fact that our next scheduled meeting probably wouldn't come off as planned—there were just too many factors that could thwart us. My bus could break down. His bus could break down. One of us could have diarrhea, or vomiting, or both. A sinkhole could open in the road. A canal could burst, flooding his village. He could *forget*. With no way to communicate, I just had to hope. But it always worked out, and that is destiny enough.

My very first inkling that I could—or would—someday get pregnant happened while we were sitting around in an apartment with a bunch of fellow rowdy Americans, drinking vodka and engaging in loud conversation that somehow ended up on the topic of pregnancy. On alcohol-induced impulse, I went over to the full-length mirror in the corner of the room, stuffing a large, roundish pillow up my shirt. Feeling tipsy, I rested my hands on my fake prego-belly and examined my reflection. *So this is what I'd look like.*

Someone saw me and shouted from across the room in a slurred voice, "You'd make a great mom, Monica!"

Embarrassed, I laughed and yanked the pillow out, glancing over at Kevin to see if he'd overheard the whole exchange, hoping that it might plant the idea in his brain that we should get married. It wasn't that I really wanted kids, not then anyway; for me, a pregnant belly was just a euphemism for eternal love. I didn't think he had witnessed my fake pregnant belly until later that night, as we were falling asleep in each other's arms on the cold, thinly carpeted floor of our friend's apartment.

"Mon?" he whispered.

"Mmm?"

"I love you. Promise we'll stay together and have an adventurous life."

I turned up to face him, and we kissed for several quiet minutes. "I love you too, but you already know that. And sure, we can keep having adventures. What should we do after Peace Corps? Manhattan?"

"Okay. Manhattan."

That's how easy it was to be with this man, how in sync we were.

Returning from Uzbekistan still dirty and unshaven, we tied the knot with a loud blow-out party at a beer garden, and spent the next five years bouncing from India to Thailand to Texas to East Africa and back, taking whatever work we could find. Eventually, we were offered dual positions teaching English to rich Saudi Arabian students in Arkansas—"Arabs in the Ozarks," as Kevin put it. It sounded different, so we went. The hilly town of Fayetteville didn't seem half bad and we quickly moved into a bright yellow rented house, just a stone's throw from the local Harley Davidson bike shop. So rural and kitschy, I know!

One evening before we had hardly unpacked boxes, I slipped into those infamous Christmas g-string panties—just because. We grilled steaks for dinner, sat on the porch swing and drank beer, talking about how strange it was that we were here now, after all these years of living in exotic places overseas. Arkansas. I didn't say "I love you," even though that's what I was thinking, because we had mutually concluded a long time ago that "I love you" was a corny thing to say. Instead, I told him I liked the way his jaw line looked in the moonlight, and we went inside and had sex on the orange futon.

And boom: the fetus had begun.

And with it, something else—that extra little bit of intangible magic that accompanies any wanted fetus: a new future with a bright sheen, filled with joyful imaginings of the baby to come. I pictured our new life together in this Norman Rockwell town, just me and Kevin and the baby-whatever-it-would-be, living in our cute yellow rented house near the town square, sitting on the porch swing and waving at the moderately good-looking, burly Harley guys revving their bikes across the street. Fayetteville, our Americana baby-raising homestead. Looking down and around, I felt happy to stop globetrotting for a while, and just live in this Technicolor, family-building reality for a while.

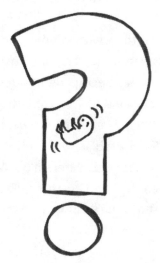

BUT NOW THAT REALITY IS GONE, right along with the fetus itself. Or himself. Or herself. Whatever. All of that—what I just said—is the most that you or I or anybody else will ever know about that little grapefruit-sized fetus, and the life of which that fetus was supposed to be front and center. Weird. One of these days, I'll wrap my head around that.

## Grandparental Love

I HONESTLY DON'T THINK parents know what to say when something like this first happens to their grown kids, especially if it's not something they've experienced themselves. It's like they suddenly feel this burst of parentalness, but they aren't sure how to channel it, since you are, after all, technically an adult who left the nest a long time ago. Here's what Mom said when she and Dad first approached me as I lay beneath a thin white hospital blanket, having lost five pounds from eating (and shitting) nothing but Popsicles: "Don't worry, honey. The baby's in heaven with Granny. She's taking good care of that little fetus."

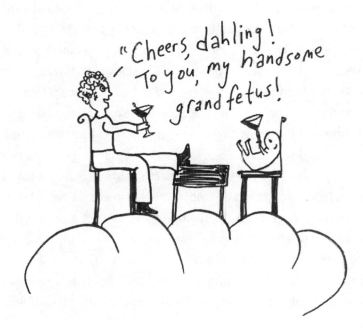

That sort of thing may have worked when I was eight or nine years old, like when we moved across the country and gave away our family dog to a "beautiful farm run by a very nice family in the mountains." It wasn't until nearly two decades later that I found out that "beautiful farm run by a very nice family in the mountains" was really a euphemism for "dog pound." A bit of a white lie, but it soothed me during those long, teary-eyed nights of missing our family pet. This time, though, such words didn't do much to soothe me, although they did generate an amusing image of Granny and Fetus sitting on a cloud top, sipping strong Manhattans together with Bing Crosby crooning in the background. That visual alone was worth it.

My parents met over thirty years ago in their early days as civil servants—IRS workers, actually, although my mom has never thought it prudent to publicize that fact—and had one child together: me. I have a half-brother named Paul, who always lived alternately with us and his hippy-photographer mother in Arizona. Paul and I finally became close when we were old enough to legally have a beer together. From a very early age, we were raised by our parents to be doers, not sit-around-and-waiters. We were always busy with sports or music, or running overseas in search of adventure. You didn't have to be especially good at what you were doing—just as long as you were doing something you enjoyed.

Nowadays, the initial miscarriage-shockwave having passed, conversations with my parents have moved to a more practical level. Mom calls several times a week, and we have the same exchange of words each time. First, she asks if there is any news about what caused the fetus to go kaput. Gotta nail down that cause, in case it's something we can prevent in the future. I always tell her the same harsh truth, knowing it isn't what she wants to hear: "They didn't pinpoint an exact cause. These things just happen—probably a chromosomal problem." Then, she asks about Kevin, and I tell her the usual: "He's fine, I guess."

More than anybody else, Mom senses when I'm not doing so well, even without my explicitly having to say so, and gently suggests various ways to move myself more clearly and proactively along the healing track.

Most of her recommendations are conventional remedies that I've already heard of, but just haven't followed through on.

The pregnancy loss support group is one such recommendation that I've resisted until now. There's one in Fayetteville for couples, but Kevin is wholly disinterested in support groups. I always tell Mom I'll give it a try, just to make her happy. For everything that Mom has done for me, the least I can do is indulge her a wee bit—even though I know deep down that I'll never be one of *those* people, the type who needs a support group.

The thing is, I like having her keeping an eye on me every week. It means a lot to know my family is there, even as the rest of the world seems to spin away.

# REVELING IN THE FETAL GLORY OF THE FETUS

FINE. I DECIDE TO TRY IT, but just this once.

Kevin opts to stay home and grease the chains of his bicycle.

"Are you sure you want to do this?" he says. "I mean, sit around with a bunch of weepy women talking about the crappiness of their situations? Might make things worse, not better."

"I think I should go just to see what it's like."

He makes me promise I'll call him on my cell phone when it's over, as though I'm about to enter some potentially dangerous carnival ride. I hop in the car and crank up "Free Bird" on the radio, drumming my fingers against the steering wheel as I cruise up the interstate. Who knows? This could be fun! I might even make some new girlfriends tonight. Not that I can imagine anyone else actually *being* at this event. What percentage of Fayetteville's few inhabitants could possibly have expelled a dead fetus in the past few months, and of *that* thin sliver of the female population, how many will have decided to attend this particular support group on this particular night? Still, surely there will be handful of likeminded participants.

I arrive fashionably late at an old Victorian house on the outskirts of town, a kind of retreat center. A fifty-something, pear-shaped woman with long graying hair and thick glasses, apparently the group facilitator, is standing at the door to greet me. We shake hands and exchange names, and I instantly forget hers, which is something nondescript like Mary or Marge. She ushers me into a cozy room full of overstuffed armchairs, where another older, gray-haired woman is casually flipping through an issue of *Woman's Day* magazine. She smiles thinly at me as I plop down into a chair beside her.

I seriously hope we aren't the only ones here. The others must have gone to the restroom.

"Well, looks like this is it, so let's get started!" says the facilitator cheerily. "My name's Marge, like I said, and this here is Candace. Monica, you go first. Go ahead! Tell us your story."

Damn. I knew it.

"Well, let's see," I begin. "A few months ago, I had a miscarriage. I was four months along. That's about it."

"Boy or girl?" says Marge. "And what did you name this precious angel, if you don't mind me asking?"

Both women are watching me expectantly. I feel my face getting hot.

"We didn't, um, ask about the gender. And we didn't give it a name."

The two women nod silently, their smiles fading. I stare down at my lap and then look back up, feeling like a schoolgirl who just gave the incorrect answer. "So anyway, that's my story. What about you guys?"

Their eyes remain on me for a second longer.

"Well," says Marge, "I've never had a miscarriage, but I'm a social worker, and I've met a lot of young ladies just like you. Candace? What about you?" She turns to face the other woman.

"I've never been through anything like this either. I'm a nurse practitioner in labor and delivery, and I've been assigned to help Marge run the group."

I guess I'm not going to make any girly new friendships tonight. Nope: just me sitting here in what feels like the hot seat, with two old ladies staring at my face. Arkansas suddenly feels even more sparsely populated than I originally thought. This whole miscarriage-having experience, in fact, is feeling sparsely populated right now.

I awkwardly stare at my lap, waiting for someone else to say something. Marge begins telling stories of past participants in the group and the kinds of beautiful burials *they* had for *their* fetuses, noting how important it is to look at the fetus, hold the fetus, play with the fetus, name the fetus, put a picture of the fetus on your desk at work, talk about the fetus every day. Good for emotional closure, Candace cuts in. But not to worry, Marge tells me, perhaps sensing my growing discomfort with the direction of this conversation: it's not too late for me to give my a fetus a name, she says, perhaps even draw a picture of what he or she *might*

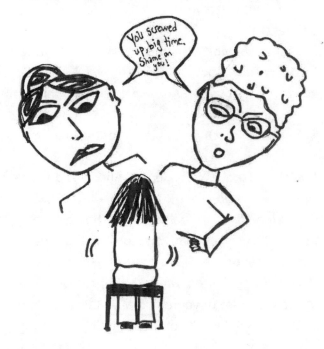

have looked like. All I can think is, *What if I don't* want *to suddenly start calling the fetus some unisex name like Pat or Jerry, or draw fetal sketches in a notebook?*

I begin to feel claustrophobic, caught blindsided in preachy conversation, as though I've been roped into an Amway sales scheme. When Marge finally suggests that I do a fake burial with a plastic doll, I glance dramatically at the clock and announce that I have…um…a coffee date to go to. Yeah, a coffee date. With a friend. Which is a hurtful lie to tell. What I wouldn't give for a *real* coffee date with a real-life girlfriend who gets it, who understands what it's like to go from pregnant to nonpregnant when you least expect it, who can help me recalibrate my mental world to the balanced, happy state it once was. I stand up to go, and Marge hands me a pastel yellow pamphlet; it's got pictures of angels on it and a phone number for a company that makes fetus-burial boxes etched with crosses. I tell her thanks, and nearly trip over myself as I dash out the front door.

"Well?" says Kevin on the phone as I sit breathlessly in the car. "How was it?"

"Sucked. I am so not cut out for this miscarriage-having thing. Oh, and apparently we fucked this whole thing up from the very beginning, so we're probably psychologically screwed forever. We were supposed to…like…revel in the fetal glory of the fetus, and we didn't. Just warning you."

"Whatever. C'mon home and drive carefully. I'm ready for Tiny Tim's."

The next day, I e-mail Mom and tell her I tried the support group, so she knows I'm not sitting around doing nothing.

# IN SEARCH OF GOD...OR SOMETHING

"WE SHOULD TRY THAT UNITARIAN CHURCH tomorrow morning."

Kevin and I are squished together on a wrought iron bench just off Dixon Street, scraping the last remnants of chocolate gelato out of paper cups. A typically benign Saturday night in Fayetteville.

"Hmm." Kevin sucks on his spoon. "What for?"

"I don't know," I say. "It just seems like church could be...a good thing at a time like this. Maybe it'll lead to some kind of spiritual epiphany for one of us. Besides, Unitarian church isn't like real church. It's more, like, people who get together for a sense of community."

"We already have a sense of community. Why don't we sleep in and screw instead?"

After my sufficient pestering, we reach a compromise: sleep in, screw, and then attend the late service. The next morning—after sleeping in and screwing—we walk to church and sit in the back row as I assured Kevin we would, a safe distance from the crowds, with easy access to an exit route.

The main speaker is a woman with long dark braids and a wrinkled face. She talks at length about living on a farm in the countryside, about her flock of chickens getting attacked by coyotes, and the spiritual lessons she learned from that experience. I concentrate on her words, trying to extrapolate some meaning that somehow relates to my miscarriage. Instead, though, I find myself thinking about chicken in a fried sense, and my stomach begins to audibly growl. I sneak a sidelong glance at Kevin, who is watching the speaker, and wonder if he's getting something from this that I'm not. The woman finishes her story, and everybody pulls little music booklets from the backs of the pews and immediately begins to sing. We frantically search for the lyrics, but by the time we find what looks like the right page, the singing is already finished.

"Now, please greet your neighbors!" says the woman, and we both reach out and awkwardly introduce ourselves to the elderly strangers around us, shaking their hands while piano music blasts in the background. I know this is probably my golden opportunity to generate that "sense of community" I was all excited about before, but instead it just feels mildly uncomfortable. To my relief, the service ends shortly thereafter, and we all stream out into the sunshine like cattle being released into the pasture.

Kevin and I duck into a café and ask if they have anything involving fried chicken, but they don't. So we settle on boring mozzarella-and-tomato sandwiches instead. After swallowing my first mouthful, I ask Kevin if he had any noteworthy epiphanies during sermon.

"Yeah," he says. "Keeping chickens sounds like a pain in the ass."

And that's it—the first and last time we set foot in a church. It was a nice thought, anyway. I call my mom that night and tell her we tried it, just in case she's writing this stuff down in a little notebook.

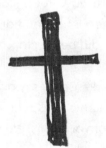

# WHEN ALL ELSE FAILS, RUN AWAY

SOMETHING IS MAKING ME FEEL ANTSY. I've felt this sensation before, the pulsating, urgent need to physically pack up and go somewhere. Kevin knows the feeling too, for it's one of the shared senses that brought us together, that has propelled us both overseas countless times in our lives, that brought us to Fayetteville in the first place.

Rural Arkansas: it seemed like a good idea at first, an adventure. But now, just five or six months after our arrival, I can't shake the itching desire to run away. I'm tired of my sulky Saudi student faces. The town feels devoid of human life, the mom-n-pop grocery store coated in a film of dust. Our little yellow house with the porch swing, what seemed like a romantic place to raise a baby, now just feels old and sagging. Fish pond dried up, yard becoming rapidly overgrown with weeds. Even the Harley Davidson shop, which used to be mildly interesting to observe from our porch, is altogether too loud. Loud dudes in leather pants that no longer look as cute as they did before, loud motorcycle sounds, loud everything.

"I think we should leave Arkansas," I say one evening, shouting over the chorus of revving engines across the street. We're sitting on the porch swing, swatting mosquitoes from our arms. Which reminds me: I'm sick of the bugs here, too.

"When? Like, now?" he yells back.

"Well yeah! Now! Like, ASAP!" I'm practically shrieking.

Kevin waits until the revving stops. "I think we need to give it at least a year."

I sigh. "But...this place just...bugs me. The bugs here bug me. There's something about it. We need to get outta here."

I know, I know. Kevin doesn't even have to remind me, because I can read his thoughts: it was half my idea to move to this tiny foreign town without a pulse, and take these teaching stints that I knew paid next to nothing. I should give it a chance, own up to my decision to come here, quit pining after something better. I know all the rationale for not upping and moving away, but rationality is not my main concern, so instead I shove my hands underneath my thighs and stare down at my lap like a sulky child.

"Well, if you can find us something better, I could maybe go for it," Kevin says, to my utter surprise. I was figuring I'd have to work harder at this one. "But it'd better be a really freakin' great job that pays a *lot* more, in an awesome location. And then that's it—we're not moving again. Not for another five years at least."

"Really??!!" I throw my arms around his torso and bury my face in his armpit, instantly flooded with hope and relief. "Aieeeeeeee! We're gettin' outta heeeeeeerrrre!"

"Calm down," he says through what I can tell is a smile, even though I'm not looking directly at his face. "It hasn't happened yet. Don't forget, it'd better be someplace worth going to."


I WASTE NO TIME IN PUTTING THIS PLAN into action. This streak of wanderlust runs deep, and isn't going to go away like the brain cancer symptoms did. Within a week, I've coaxed Kevin into applying for a job near Seattle, teaching computer classes to prisoners (yes, real prisoners who do bad things and spend their lives behind bars). Seattle is perfect for us, I assure him, populated and civilized and blessed with lovely gray skies under which to raise a family, and mountains to hike in. We'll be all cozy and wearing sweaters and playing Scrabble next to the fireplace. No more sweat rashes on the inner thighs, no more bugs, no more revving Harley engines!

Kevin soon gets offered the job and calls to accept it. From that point forward, everything moves at a rapid and giddy pace. Within a month, we've packed our increasingly slimmed-down collection of belongings into boxes ("three moves is as good as a fire," as our friend Henry says, which means that chronic nomads like us end up with the bare bones minimum), and said moderately emotional goodbyes to the small group of friends and acquaintances we've accumulated through the language school. We then make the multi-day slog to Seattle in a small U-Haul truck, stopping overnight in Vegas to see my parents, who are there to play quarter slots. They both tell me separately that it's good to see us looking so excited. An astute observation, because I *am* excited. This finally feels like progress toward something.

In the middle of the night, both clutching our Styrofoam cups half-full of gas-station coffee, we finally pass a green freeway sign that reads, "Entering Seattle." The windshield wipers can barely keep up with the driving rain, and big, black hills loom up around us, dotted with lights. The landlord at our new apartment is waiting for us with a wet key, which we grab excitedly from his hands with hardly a hello. We brush right past him and race out the sliding glass doors onto the rooftop deck.

I weave my fingers through Kevin's and we stand huddled together, looking out over the city skyline as raindrops dampen our hair and face. I take a deep breath of nighttime air through my nose; it smells of woody wetness, vaguely piney…of water running down concrete and between tree roots. I did live here until I was ten years old, so I suppose I should recognize this city, these scents—but I don't. Instead, I am buzzing with that surreal, woundrous feeling of landing in a foreign country, of seeing a place for the very first time. It's the smell of a fresh start, a new life, a chance to try again for a real, bona fide baby. I know it will happen, now that the perplexing and still-aching memories of decaying goldfish and our lost fetus have been left behind. A feeling—for the first time in months—of being alive.

Which means, hopefully, that I can take a break from running for a while. Chill out, and just live. And maybe even bust out that g-string again, if I can find it. I think I might be ready for it.

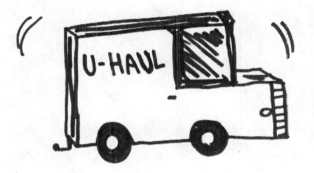

# The Second Journey Segment:
## From an Urban Oasis of Love, Hope, and Purposeful Sex

*January to August, 2007*

# When You Don't Make the Cheerleading Squad

WE KNOW EXACTLY TWO PEOPLE upon arriving in Seattle: Jane and Jayson, a married couple we befriended in Austin five years ago. Jane's had a miscarriage too, and for that I feel a special connection to her. We'll become best buddies and start an exclusive anti-pregnancy club out of spite, calling ourselves the Knocked-Up-Knocked-Downers! We'll look at pregnant women with wistful disdain, have secret handshakes, and wear goth hairstyles and black t-shirts that say, *"We didn't want babies anyway. So screw you, world!"* Plus, she's got a tattoo like me. (Mine is a relic of drunk-n-high night in college, not the result of anything meaningful). Perfect.

Jane quickly e-mails to invite us over for dinner. Homecoming time! Break out the wine and checkered tablecloth—time to get drunk and gorge ourselves with old friends who share a common miserable experience! Brag about how much our lives suck! Commiserate about our respective dead fetuses! Make fun of support groups! Then I get to the second half of her message, where she tells me she's pregnant and due in just a few months, and my stomach lurches down a few notches. I can hear that horn of disappointment going "wahh wahhhhhhh" inside my head.

So much for our anti-baby club.

I feel crestfallen, abandoned by I don't know what, and then ashamed for feeling that way. After chewing fretfully on my fingernails for a moment, I decide to suck it up and respond the way Mom would want me to if Jane had gotten into the cheerleading squad and I hadn't, for that's kind of how this feels.

"Jane, that is AWESOME!" I type, hoping the all-caps isn't overkill. "I'm SOOO happy for you. See you tonight."

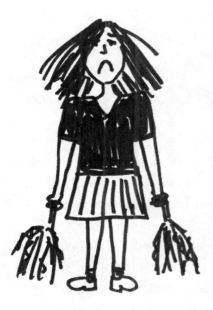

After hitting "send," I sidle up next to Kevin, who is sitting on the futon, his nose in a copy of *Maxim*. He appears to be reading an informational blurb about a bikini-clad brunette I don't recognize, although I can't tell if he's paying more attention to the blurb or the close-up shot of her cleavage.

"Jane's pregnant," I say, pseudo-offhandedly.

"Oh," he says, his eyes flickering up from the page for a split second, and then drifting back down to the text blurb. Or the cleavage beside the text blurb. Whatever.

That's it: just plain *oh*.

I watch him for several seconds longer, to see if there might be more to that sentence, but there isn't. With a flash of exasperation, I wonder why men (and with Kevin, I feel honestly okay with equating his behavior to most men in the world, because he's such a typical guy-guy) are so incapable of understanding the deeper ramifications of such things. *Jane's pregnant*.

Exasperation quickly morphs into a different, worse concern: perhaps the problem is *me*, not Kevin or Jane or anyone else. Maybe there are no deeper ramifications, and I'm making this into a big, unnecessary mess. God, what is WRONG with me? Where is the joy that this kind of news is supposed to bring to a person? *I* certainly expected people to be nothing short of ecstatic when they found out *I* was pregnant, so why should Jane and her baby deserve anything less? I ponder how I became this sort of subhuman life form, incapable of feeling glad about my friend's good fortune. Everyone except me apparently sees things in a sane and normal way. I decide to drop the subject.

THAT NIGHT, WE DRIVE ALONG the city's windy roads, up and down hills and over majestic bridges to the upscale neighborhood of Montlake, pulling up in front of Jane and Jayson's rented house. As we approach the front door, it swings open before we have the chance to knock. Jane is standing there waving and smiling from ear to ear, light brown hair pulled away from her face in a ponytail. Her belly, which is as enormous as mine should have been a few months back, is proudly visible from beneath her form-fitting white maternity top. There is a knot in the core of my torso.

"Hiiiiiiii! So great to see you!" We exchange big hugs, and Jane is visibly glowing as she takes my coat. Jayson, chatting amicably, leads us on a brief tour of the house, which is brimming with big, expensive-looking wooden furniture and framed artwork. The baby room is totally set up with a new crib and area rug and dresser, all of it still smelling like a department store. Everywhere, clear markings of financial and reproductive success.

"Can I pop open some wine for anyone?" Jayson asks.

"ME!" I say a little too loudly and quickly. There are no other takers, and I feel momentarily self-conscious about this fact, but let it go. Hell—if I'm going to be the sulky one with the fake smile, I'd rather do it buzzed than sober.

Kevin and I have remarked in the past that with these particular friends, it always ends up like this: the men in one area of the house, talking about stereotypically male things like politics and gadgets, and the women in another area of the house, discussing food and clothing and the gossipy secrets of mutual acquaintances. Tonight is no exception. Kevin and Jayson settle into the living room sofa, conversing about how universally crappy the U-Haul company is, while I stand in the kitchen and sip (or rather, gulp) my cold white wine, watching Jane take thick spinach-and-Fontina-cheese stuffed pork chops out of the oven. I ask Jane if I can help with anything, and she says no. Moving gingerly, careful not to bang her bulging belly on the edge of the counter top, she tells me she's been eating full fat organic everything lately. Kind of pricey, she notes, but totally worth it. I swirl my wine around in my glass and chug the remainder of it, taking the liberty of pouring myself a refill. My thoughts are starting to slur together.

Finally, we all sit down to eat at the long table in the dining room, which feels like a Crate and Barrel showroom—complete with matching cloth napkins, sparkling silverware and wine glasses, and flickering candles. The conversation bounces cheerfully between benign topics—the details of Jayson's consulting job, old memories from when we all lived in Austin together—remaining safely distant from dead fetuses, or anything else baby-related for that matter (although I vaguely, sadistically wish that unwanted subject would arise). Jane brings out a triple-layer carrot cake, perfectly tall and cylindrical and slathered with white frosting, a model cake for the cover of *Good Housekeeping*. We eat more than our stomachs can really hold, smothering Jane and her food with compliments. As the chatter slows and becomes sleepy, we all stand up, and Jane and Jayson graciously thank us for coming over.

Just as we're about to walk out the door, I notice that the tattoos that used to be on the top of Jane's feet are now gone completely, leaving barely noticeable scars from laser surgery. That's it—the deal is sealed. We're not best buddies, which means I'm still stuck by myself in this strange and depressing land of knocked-up-knocked-down.

If Mom were here now, she would brush my hair off my forehead and slip into that soft and nurturing tone of voice, reminding me of all of the wonderful things I have, of how pretty and smart and talented I am, of how fortunate I've been in life. I try to imagine those words as Kevin and I climb into the chilly car, but still find myself focusing on what's missing: a real baby in my belly, not a mere memory of a faceless fetus who didn't make it. Some decent furniture and place settings, instead of a bunch of mismatched crap from garage sales and Target. The ability to bake a perfectly gorgeous, cylindrical cake, rather than the sunken rectangular variety that shows up at church bake-sales. I feel dully distraught, uncomfortably stuffed, and rummage unsuccessfully in the glove box for a spare roll of Tums. Kevin rests one hand on my thigh.

"That was fun," I say forcefully, in a half-hearted stab at good sportsmanship. "Awesome pork chops. Jane looks great, doesn't she?" There. That's the "me" that Kevin married, the sort of thing I would normally say before I turned into Miss Negative.

"Yeah," says Kevin, glancing in my direction for a split second. "So, you did okay with Jane being pregnant and all?"

I pause for a moment, looking out my window as I feel my eyebrows furrow in the middle. "I'm okay. The wine helped."

I'm okay. Maybe the key to feeling it is to say it enough times.

# A ROCKY MOVIE MONTAGE

I WAKE UP TO THE SOOTHING SOUNDS of coffee percolating and Kevin padding about the kitchen in his socks, opening and closing drawers. A rare ray of morning sun is shining through the small window above the stairwell, casting a square of light on the opposite wall; I can see it from where my head is positioned on the pillow. I flip the covers off and sit up, stretching and yawning, making a loud "ahhhhhh!" sound.

This is it: a brand new day, time to roll up my sleeves and get busy putting my life in order, the way it was a long time ago, back when I used to be a sexy and productive human being. I put on my moose slippers, go into the kitchen, and kiss Kevin on his sandpapery neck.

"Hey."

"Hey."

After microwaving myself half a mug of milk and topping it off with coffee, I settle into the couch with the laptop balanced on my knees.

"We need three things, Kev. The first is, I have to score a full-time job. That's going to be my focus this week, starting today."

"I would agree with that."

"Ready for the next thing?"

"Sure."

"We need a social life. That's going to be my secondary focus."

"I don't know how much of a social life you can expect after living in a new city for…what…five days. Anyway, what about Jane and Jayson? Last time I checked, they counted as friends."

"Yeah, but Jane's, you know. So I can't be hanging out with her all the time—that won't work for a variety of reasons. Ready for the third thing?"

"Sure. Hold that thought—I gotta take a piss." He goes into the bathroom and closes the door.

I've never been one to wait around for things like pissing. "A BABY!" I yell. This is too important to hold inside. "WE NEED A BABY TO MAKE UP FOR THAT LAST ONE! WE NEED ONE SO WE CAN GET AHEAD IN LIFE!"

"We're already having sex, aren't we?" he calls out from behind the closed bathroom door, his voice muffled.

"YEAH, BUT OBVIOUSLY NOT ENOUGH! WE NEED TO START MAKING IT A POINT TO SCREW A LOT MORE, BUT ONLY AT NIGHT, JUST BEFORE BED, SO I CAN BE LYING DOWN FOR EIGHT HOURS AND YOUR SPERM WON'T TRICKLE OUT! I'LL EVEN START WEARING THAT G-STRING AGAIN, IF I CAN FIND IT!"

For a fleeting instant, I wonder if the neighbors can hear me shouting. Even if they can, who cares? I doubt we'll be living here for long. Soon I'll have a job that pays me decent money and a new baby growing inside of me, and we'll buy a house to celebrate. A real house of our own: the final component necessary in order to have *a real life*. As I gaze out the window, fantasizing about babies and houses and jobs, I hear the toilet flush and water running for a few seconds, and the bathroom door opens. Kevin plops down next to me and puts his hand on my thigh, leaning in toward my ear.

"Fine with me. We could do a quickie right now, even."

I glance up at him from my laptop screen. Didn't we just decide that morning sex isn't a part of the plan? Then I realize I'm planning too much and not really living. Living, I remind myself, is still being able to arouse a man after nearly five years of marriage. So I gulp down the rest of my coffee and set the computer aside.

"All right," I say, nuzzling his nose with mine.

RUNNING ON THIS SUDDEN INFUSION of inspiration, life becomes movie montage with me as the sweaty and determined star, bold and hope-filled Rocky theme music in the background. At least, that's how I see it. My goal, simply put, is to construct a satisfactory reality in Seattle, complete with an admirably extensive set of friends, a job for me, and a child. I attack this multi-pronged task with gusto, pleased to have a set of objectives to work toward, a renewed sense of control over my own destiny.

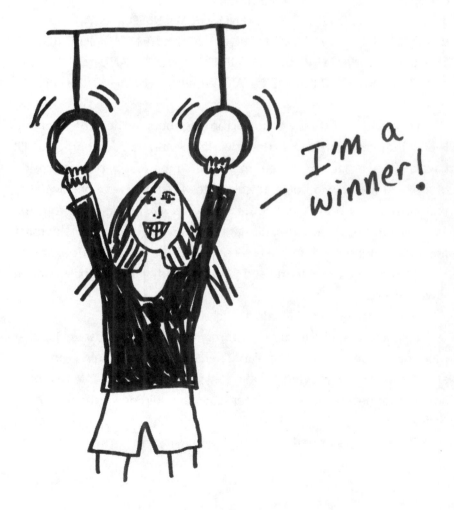

I e-mail my mom to preemptively assure her that everything is falling into place. She's glad to hear it, she writes, reminding me once more to keep her posted on any news about what caused the miscarriage. I wish she weren't so hung up on that mysterious detail. It's cramping my style, this lingering concern about that dark spot on my past, forcing me to think about an event that I'd just as soon forget. *That's just how moms are,* I remind myself.

Kevin begins teaching weeknights at the prison, thus initiating our new Seattle routine. He seems pleased with the work that he's doing, unconcerned about working with felons, just—as usual—fine. Admittedly, I didn't realize—in my crazed rush to get us out of Arkansas—that this new job would keep him away until ten o'clock on most nights. To fill the void of being home by myself after dark, I pick up a few evening English classes to teach at a local college. Kevin prints out maps and marks the best cycling routes for me with a ballpoint pen, and with newfound confidence, I begin traveling from gig to gig on my bike, something I've never done before.

Despite the near-constant drizzle, I enjoy my open-air commute with the wind on my face, the vibrant city sights and sounds swirling around me. Everything feels alive and civilized compared to empty, quiet Fayetteville. Vibrant blocks of shops with living people meandering inside them! Cars and people in constant motion, zipping purposefully from place to place! Bodies of blue-gray water everywhere, lakes and bays and sounds, joined by even more water. Old, colorful neighborhoods carved into the forest green hillsides, connected by soaring bridges. It feels refreshingly like a pulsating, breathing place where life happens.

In the mornings, I spend hours putting together application packets for full-time teaching positions that start in the fall, just as a back-up plan in case I'm not a mother by then. And every night, in preparation for my calculated pre-bedtime sexual attack on Kevin, I shower and shave and tousle my hair—skipping the lotion and deodorant because I know he prefers the taste of skin unadulterated by such chemical products. Fortunately, he doesn't seem to mind my forceful and frequent demands for intercourse. (For the record, I don't feel quite ready to bust out the g-string just yet, so I go about my baby-making efforts without them, hoping to ride some of the leftover g-string energy from the last time I wore them nearly a year ago. Besides, I still haven't found them from whatever bin of clothing they were haphazardly shoved into.)

Meanwhile, I busily begin simulating a social life. We join the local Peace Corps alumi group and get introduced to a "childfree by choice" couple: Bruce—an environmental something-or-other for the county, and Carrie—a former pastry chef now studying naturopathic medicine, thin and blond but in a warm and earthy sort of way. Right away, I fall in love with them, their relaxed marriedness and purposeful childlessness, their cozy little house with mismatched furniture and a cabinet full of hard liquor, the fact that they both worked on Alaskan fishing boats. Soon after meeting them, I insist that they come over for dinner, ignoring Kevin's suggestion that one night without social plans might be nice. The four of us sit around the kitchen island and drink strong Bombay and tonics with extra lime, gnawing on the garlic cheddar biscuits that I made in an attempt to mimic the ones from Red Lobster, only to have them mysteriously turn hard as bricks. But the booze and conversation flow with such animated ease that nobody seems to notice. Again, I shoot Kevin that *happiness* look, because happiness and hope are what I feel.

# FETUS MORPHING

MY MEDICAL RECORDS ARRIVE from Fayetteville, a thick paper-clipped stack inside of a manila envelope. I've never looked at these before, so of course I'm instantly intrigued. Kevin slides the envelope underneath a stack of bills and magazines on the dining room table, presumably hoping this will keep me from perusing them with fascination. I have a sudden image of him ahead of me on this road to somewhere, armed and scouting for pitfalls with the keen eye of a Marine Corps colonel's son, which he is. Watching for dangers that might make me lose my footing and regress into a state of gloominess, and kicking them off to the side where they won't harm me.

I'm not saying it's wrong of him to think like this, by the way. Once the fetus is gone, isn't the wife the only thing remaining? He's got to keep her intact, protect her at all costs. It comes from his family, too: *is Monica okay?* That's how phone calls with his parents, two brothers, and sister began during the days and weeks following the incident, and now it's how they always end. Lingering concern: *is Monica okay?* Everyone seems more comfortable when Monica—and therefore Kevin—is okay.

Going back to those medical records, calling my name from under the stack of mail: Kevin is probably right. Unearthing this sordid piece of medical history does seem distinctly counterproductive. Who knows how much shockingly gory detail they reveal about that fateful day, which exact adjectives they use to describe our partially formed baby and its various accoutrements, what sort of painful and grotesque image they will conjure up.

57

But that envelope beckons me like a giant chocolate cupcake set in front of a hungry woman on a diet. I briefly consider sneaking a glance at the envelope's contents while Kevin is asleep; I could hide them behind the newspaper in case he woke up, pretending to be doing some late-night scanning of the employment section. But instead I decide to read them here and now, right out in the open. Changing into my sweats and a t-shirt, I open a fresh jar of Clausen dills, pull out those records, and settle into the sofa to give them a good look-over while chomping on a pickle.

"Sure you wanna see those?" Kevin glances over his shoulder from his dish-washing position in front of the sink.

"Yeah, yeah. Just, ya know. Curious. It's not like I don't already know what they're going to say."

Kevin doesn't come over to read them with me, but turns back to the sink. He apparently doesn't have the same masochistic desire to pelt himself with depressing reminders. I bite into a pickle and open the thick, stapled packet to a random page in the middle.

*06-30-06. Patient presents for new OB care at 15 ½ weeks gestation. Fetal heart tones are absent, and abdominal ultrasound was undertaken. There is no evidence of cardiac activity or evidence of fetal movement. This was felt to represent an intrauterine fetal demise.*

Harmless enough so far; nothing I haven't heard. I skip ahead a few pages, hoping to get to the gross part. Finally, amidst the boring medical terminology, a phrase pops out abruptly like a flashing blue light: "male fetus." I skip up a line to read that phrase once more: "male fetus." Yup, I read that correctly.

"It was gonna be a boy," I hear myself say tautly, my mouth still half full of pickle.

Long pause from Kevin. "Hmmm. That's what the records say?"

"Yeah. Male fetus. It says that right here. I guess that's not…something we ever knew. The gender, I mean."

Kevin loudly scrubs a greasy pot, glancing over in my direction. I set down the envelope and walk into the bathroom, shutting the door behind me. Once there, I plop down onto the fake wood floor beside the ceramic toilet bowl, and bury hands in my face, feeling like a child who just got punched at recess. In this case, punched by myself, since I'm the one that insisted on opening that envelope. With my hands pressed against my closed eyes, the summer memory of 2006 floods back for the first time in months, a string of images stored beneath my skin now pushing out through my pores.

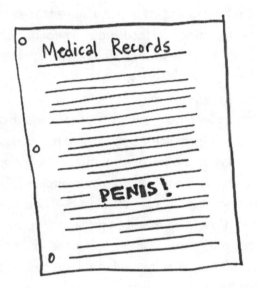

I see a dimly lit ultrasound screen, with an intense clarity of detail that almost feels as though I've returned there, jumped backward in time. It's like one of those mosaic dot posters that were popular back in the day, the ones where you had to focus your eyes just right in order to see the hidden image. When I concentrate hard enough, I can see something that looks distinctly baby-like, curled up appropriately in fetal position, with its spindly arms and legs, small as twigs, and disproportionately large head. A shrunken version of a real baby, frozen perfectly still, floating in a sac of amniotic fluid.

I ask the doctor how he knows for certain that this floating little fetus is not alive. Not that I don't trust his expertise, but this cruelly shocking announcement is so far off the map that I feel I'm owed an explanation. The heart was just beating at my appointment a week earlier, I remind him with as steady a voice as I can muster. Even the nurse can vouch for this. But he simply points to the screen and tells me gently, but with conviction, that the heart of a nearly four-month fetus should look like a great big butterfly flapping its wings. I stare at that screen for a long period of silence, squinting and focusing and refocusing, sensing that I'm the only non-believer in the room. Kevin rests his hands on my forearm and breathes quietly, not saying a word. Waiting, maybe, for me to get it. Or perhaps he's also stunned speechless.

Finally, with a sweeping mental shift, I concede that I don't see the butterfly at all, let alone its wings flapping, and feel as though a guillotine just sliced me in half at the torso. Pain: physical, wind-knocking pain, a raw and disorienting new emotion, utterly unfamiliar. I cover my face with my hands and begin to cry harder than I've ever cried before, the heavy and silent kind that could be mistaken for laughing, and the doctor and nurses file quietly out of the room and shut the door. Kevin is there for me fiercely and fully as usual, gathering me up so that I'm leaning into his chest and holding me there with his arms. I am limp and heaving like a rag doll with a violent case of the hiccups, and can hardly summon the strength to remain upright. Everything in my world sort of flattens out and turns gray.

That memory vanishes, replaced by an image of myself days later, lying in a pool of blood in the emergency ward with people hovering around me. Kevin is there, of course. Somebody says "push" and I do, and then something slippery and three-dimensional flies out of me, and it's all over. Kevin's slightly red-rimmed eyes are trained on my face, and I feel exhausted and relieved as I bring my knees together, allowing them to lean on one another. Relieved that my husband is there, keeping track of me. Fleetingly, I hope he's doing okay.

"Don't look down, Kev," I say, suddenly terrified that he might see it, this semi-developed, baby-like entity covered in bodily fluids, a sight that could very well haunt him for the rest of his life. He nods and whispers that he won't look, still gazing directly into my eyes. Goodness, I love this man.

Fast forward to now, as I sit just inches from a gleaming white toilet seat.

Now, for the first time ever, instead of a baby-like entity covered in bodily fluids, I see a *child* behind the reddish blackness of my closed eyelids. An infant with dark brown hair and a tiny little penis, morphing into a thumb-sucking toddler and then a bright and wide-eyed adolescent boy in quick succession, his growth stopping there. He looks almost like a drawing from a children's book, cartoonish and perfect, with a smattering of freckles on his face and a slightly sunburned nose beneath the rim of his baseball cap. *A boy.* I hear the *thunk* of water shutting off in the kitchen, and then Kevin's soft voice outside the bathroom door.

"Mon?"

"Mmm?" I hardly recognize my own voice, an anguished squeak.

Kevin comes inside, pulling me to my feet. "C'mere, let's go lie down."

My hands stay plastered on my face, grief sucking everything I've got inward, like a gigantic vacuum. I'm relieved to have somebody directing me, and hope for the hundredth time that I'm not taking too much, that this residual grief isn't overstaying its welcome in our marriage, that I didn't push the envelope too far by diving into those records. I clamor up onto the bed, flopping down on my backside. Kevin comes up too, sliding up next to me.

"I think it's that I miss him," I say up to the ceiling. "He was going to be our kid."

"I know you miss him. So do I."

"He had a lot of potential. He was going to look like you. He would have been…what, a month old by now? In five years or whatever, you'd be showing him how to hit a whifle ball with one of those big red plastic bats."

"Yeah." Kevin's body tenses. We lie this way for a long time, until my tears and snot are all dried up and I've nothing left to feel. I blow my nose on the corner of pillowcase, while Kevin discreetly grabs a handful of toilet paper off the bedside table and places it into my hand.

"Do you still think I'm sexy?" I ask into his armpit, knowing it's another feminine and needy question, but craving his "yes" anyway, because hearing that answer is like sinking my teeth into warm homemade chicken potpie on a cold winter day. Comforting.

He sits up and brushes my bangs out of my eyes, a gesture I love. "Yes."

"Can we go out for fish-n-chips?" I say.

"Sure. Let's go."

We walk five blocks uphill to the Blue Star and sit at the dimly lit bar, ordering two amber beers and a platter of fried cod to share. I dump salt on my half of the fish before taking a bite, while Kevin squirts a zigzag line of ketchup across his half of fries. We talk about our jobs, about traveling to China in December, and I'm relieved to feel more or less normal again. *Cleansed of feeling*, for now anyway. It's funny how we get these bouts of emotion out of our system, and then slip back into relative normalcy so easily.

"Are you okay?" I ask, not because I have any doubt that he's okay, but because it makes me feel like our relationship is on an even keel. Like we're taking care of each other—not just him of me. A team project. "I mean, in terms of...you know."

"I'm okay, but I need you to be okay too."

That's it: a concise, straight-up honest answer a la Kevin. It's the first time I've heard him say this in the six months since the fetus left us. See? I knew my husband-as-armed-scout analogy wasn't too far off the mark. I down the remainder of my beer, setting down my glass, and gaze past Kevin at the flickering reflections of people's silhouettes in the mirror behind the bar. In a moment of crystal clarity and certitude, I understand exactly what I need to do: *be okay.*

Not that this is the first time I've thought this exact thing. Of course, from day one I've been striving to be okay. This time it's different, though, because it isn't just for me now, but for him. *For us.* I have to give this man who does so much for me, expecting so little in return, the one thing he needs: *my okayness.* Myself, unchanged, the person he fell in love with.

"I'll be okay," I say, repeating the same mental command I've already issued to myself more times than I can count: *just be okay.*

# FREEFALL INTO JOY

EVEN THOUGH I'VE SAID WE NEED A BABY, I wouldn't exactly say I'm *in love* with the idea of snotty, poopy germ-filled offspring clamoring around my feet, getting in the way of sex and happy hour, sucking up all of my and Kevin's financial and emotional resources, dumbing down the dinner conversation. I didn't get my Master's degree so I could sit at home and watch Home Shopping Network with a pump attached to my nipple. Nope; I'm a career woman with ambitions beyond all that. Rationally, I know that becoming a mom is probably one of those things you think you want, and then once you get it, you wonder with horror what you've gotten yourself into. Still, despite all of the above, I want it. Nothing, it seems, could be more likely to catapult Kevin and me into eternal fineness than a child.

It happens late one morning like a déjà vu, after Kevin has left for work: I awaken with a dry throat and chug a gigantic glass of cold water, only to vomit the entire contents of my stomach immediately into the toilet. If it were possible to smile and throw up at the same time, I'd be doing it—because I know.

I don't bother calling Kevin, who is sequestered in a dark prison unit without cell phone service. Instead, I stride out into the glorious sunshine, hop aboard my bike, and take it for a spin through the tree-lined streets. The Space Needle and a sea of gleaming skyscrapers soar in the distance, backed by a sparkling strip of cobalt blue. Seattle is, like Fayetteville was at one time, *the perfect place to raise a baby*. And me, as a mom: *the perfect notion*. I'm flooded with the familiar feelings of anticipation, purposefulness, and clarity of mind that I've not felt since last summer.

I shove my used pee-stick in Kevin's face as he walks in the front door that night, and he reacts with measured caution, suggesting we wait a few months before announcing the news. Even though our little secret is bubbling up inside me like a thunderous burp, dying to get out, I nod my head in theoretical agreement.

I said "theoretical," right?

Four days later, Bruce and Carrie invite us over for dinner. As we sit around their cozy kitchen table, picking crumbles of cheese off a wooden cutting board, Carrie pours herself a glass of fruit punch.

"We have some unexpected news," she says. "I'm pregnant, due in October."

I breathe in sharply. Carrie, our self-proclaimed, childless-by-choice friend, *knocked up*! And knocked up *now*, of all times!

"OMIGOD," I blurt out impulsively, casting Kevin a pleadingly apologetic look. "ME TOO!!!"

We all stand up and hug, clinking glasses and oohing and ahhing over each other's marvelous news. It's mostly Carrie and me doing the chatting.

It isn't more than a few weeks later that Jane delivers her baby prematurely. It's okay now, her having a baby and all, because this month I've so moved past my earlier hang-ups with her belly, her tattoo-less-ness, her admirably arranged life. The baby shower is at Jayson's parents' sprawling, modern home in a woodsy suburban neighborhood. I make the drive by myself, since it's supposedly a ladies-only event. The high-ceilinged, sunlit living room is crammed full of clucking women, old and young, with a tired-looking Jane resting in an armchair in the corner. Baby Jeffrey is swaddled in a blanket on her lap. He is tiny, the length of my forearm, if not smaller. It's a poignant and humanizing sight, Jane with her expression of serenity and exhaustion, and without warning I am hit with a dull pang of guilt for not feeling sufficiently glad about my friend's happy pregnancy early on.

I say my hellos and hug the right people, tossing my gift in the gift pile, taking a turn at gingerly holding the feather-light infant. As

I awkwardly cradle his head in the palm of my head, I envision myself holding my own warm newborn in eight months with everybody around me celebrating, and my stomach does a little forward flip of excitement. Impulsively, I lean into Jane's ear.

"I'm pregnant again," I whisper. It somehow just seems like a cosmically appropriate time and place to tell her, even though it breaks (again) the multi-month code of secrecy that I semi-promised Kevin, and even though this event is supposed to be about Jane, not about me. Her eyes widen, a smile spreading across her face as she throws her arms around my neck.

"Oh my God! Monica! Oh my God! I am so happy for you!"

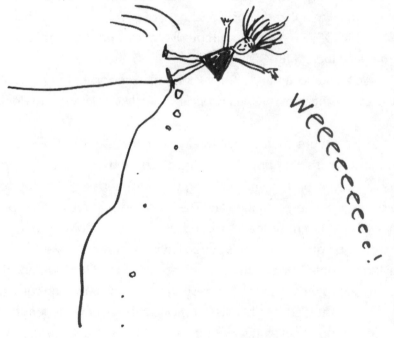

I feel connected to her, the way humans are supposed to feel. We hug tightly around Jeffrey's warm body, frozen like that for several long seconds, and I pull back and say I'll keep her posted. She sniffles and tells me she'll be in charge of the baby shower. The baby shower! I haven't even thought about that.

"I...um....told Jane," I tell Kevin that evening, kind of sorry about it, but not really. How can I not tell the world? Something momentous is happening, a baby! He cracks open a beer and looks at me, not saying a whole lot. I can sense his discomfort with all this unrestrained yapping, because—like a good scout—he sees potential danger in our pathway long before I ever do. And although these seem like simple and harmless conversations with friends, he knows it's hurling me haphazardly forward without suitable armor. But I'm already gone so he's letting me go, keeping watch as my figure gets smaller in the distance.

The funny thing is, when you're married long enough, you figure these things out about the inner workings of one another's minds. Still, you plow ahead with the role you know is yours, and trust each other to pick up the slack in your own area of shortcoming. Kevin can stay as cautious as he wants for the both of us. As for me, I'm going with what I feel.

Unfettered joy.

## Assembling a New Tribe

IT'S A CROWDED SATURDAY MORNING at the Blue Star, and throngs of people are standing and sitting, clutching menus and hungrily eyeing the waitresses. Kevin has wandered off to find the restroom while I stand near the window, scanning the crowds for anyone that seems to be scanning for me. I'm beginning to wonder if everyone bailed, if it's going to be just Kevin and me for brunch.

"Hey! Are you Monica?"

I spin around, coming face to face with a pretty, grinning girl in an army-green, form-fitting jacket, her hair—somewhere between brown and blond—pulled back off her face in an elastic headband. Right away, I like her. I like the self-assured sparkle in her blue eyes—as in, *of course you're Monica*—and, most of all, her voice. Low-pitched and loud, not timid and mousy. An articulate voice projected with confidence, like the voice of a theatre major. I wouldn't be surprised if she was a teacher like me. The best teachers have loud, commandeering voices.

"Hey! You must be Nina."

We shake hands firmly, lingering for a moment with our palms locked. Instinctively, I glance downward for a split second, searching for a perceptible bump in her bellybutton region. There isn't one, which is cool, because I don't have one either quite yet. We're in sync, and we're going to be friends. I can already tell.

Our respective husbands—alike in their dark hair, lanky tallness, and white-toothed smiles—simultaneously appear beside us, and everyone gets introduced again. *This is Kevin; this is David.* Seconds later, we are ushered to a wooden booth, collectively sighing with relief. Relief that we finally get to eat, but also—for me, anyway—relief that somebody showed up for the debut gathering of the Seattle First-Time Urban Expecting Parents Group, of which I am the official organizer. And not just any old socially inept somebody that you might get stuck with on a blind date (which is kind of what this is), forced to awkwardly make conversation while hurriedly shoving your food down your throat. Nope—Nina and David are clearly interesting people with more than adequate conversational skills.

We all order things involving bacon and cheese, and slip instantly into dynamic, profanity-laden conversation, divulging the basic details of our lives. She *is* a teacher (didn't I call it?), and he's a tech marketing guy. They first met at a college party and French kissed on the dance floor. Eventually, they moved into an apartment and raised a small Aussie-poodle mix named Rover together. Nina and I do most of the talking, our animated voices filling the booth space while Kevin and David chuckle and nod and make occasional side remarks. We then launch into our pregnancies, the exciting common thread that has brought us here in the first place, realizing with joyful astonishment that our babies are due the same week in October. I think about Carrie as we talk, about this uncanny good fortune of knowing not just one, but now *two* knocked up ladies whose babies are due within days of mine.

Nearly two hours later, long after we have all sopped up the last bits of egg yoke from our plates and begun to shift in our seats from our butts falling asleep, we stand up and exchange hearty hugs. To me, it feels as though the four of us have known each other for some time, a testimony to the power of pregnancy as a connector of people. As we walk out, Kevin pulls me toward him.

"They're going to be good friends to have," he says, and I wonder if he's feeling less guarded than before.

"I know! Weren't they just awesome? I can't believe Nina was in a sorority! She doesn't act like a sorority girl."

OTHER COUPLES JOIN OUR LITTLE GROUP, and I quickly become a mad planner of brunches and dinners and cheese-tasting outings, positioning myself eagerly as a pregnant social queen and dragging Kevin alongside. Like chameleons, Kevin and I become innocently eager first-timers—hugging and shaking hands, comparing belly sizes, tossing around baby names and the latest rumors about which prenatal vitamins are best.

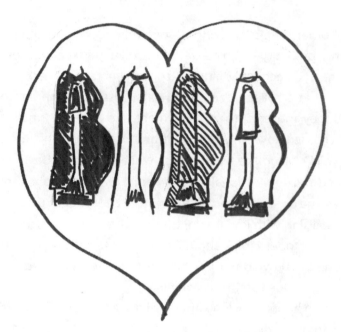

But of all the women in the club, Nina is still the one I feel closest to. It isn't only that we feed off each other's pregnant giddiness and dramatic, pseudo-fears of prenatal disaster. It isn't just the thrilling notion of raising our babies together. It isn't just that we laugh often and with gusto— usually at the exact same things—or that neither of us has qualms about conversing loudly in public about sex and poop. All of those things are a part of it, of course. But more than anything else, Nina embodies a rosy-cheeked vitality that she draws out in me (and everyone she meets, I suspect). When we're together, yammering on our cell phones, her positive energy further erases that drab, unstable, Hanes-wearing me from the Arkansas days. Not that I'm strutting around in that Christmas g-string and a lacey teddy, since we all know those naughty apparel items don't mesh with heavy pregnant bodies (and since I still can't find those long-lost panties anyway), but still. I feel refreshed, feminine, alive inside—unshackled by melancholy and paranoia—especially in the presence of Nina.

I quickly introduce her to Carrie, of course, and we get together occasionally to stroll the three-mile path around shimmering Green Lake, a tree-lined oasis in the middle of the city. Carrie brings a much-needed streak of calm to my and Nina's fast-talking, loud-laughing dynamic. Carrie knows about my ill-fated pregnancy history because I told her, sensing her earthy ability to empathize—even with things she hasn't experienced. Nina I haven't told yet. Not because it's some deep dark secret, but because I simply can't bear the thought of tugging down our buoyantly joyful friendship—founded on the buoyantly joyful premise of pending motherhood—with something so heavy and outdated. That miscarriage is so 2006. Sometimes, all that dirt from the past is best left untouched.

# PUTTING THE PIECES TOGETHER

LATELY, I'VE BEGUN TO VIEW LIFE as a puzzle comprised of a whole bunch of pieces. They all come together if you make the right choices, and—as I often remind Kevin—our big puzzle is shaping up nicely. Not bad for having only lived in Seattle for five months.

Social piece: check. No complaints in the friend department. Got our prego friends, our non-prego friends, and, of course, each other as best-of-the-best friends. All good.

The sex piece: eh, not so much. I wouldn't exactly say that random, passion-induced intercourse is high on my list these days—especially when my vagina's main function will soon involve ejecting a large, blood-covered mammal. Those sexy Christmas panties are around somewhere, I'm sure, but we all know that responsible moms—or almost-moms like me—don't wear such things. For now, I'm content with curve-swallowing Hanes and baggy maternity garbs.

The kid piece: check. See that bump rising below my belly button? The one blending in to my existing spare tire, just enough to make it look like an even bigger fat tire? Enough said.

The financial piece: check. Kevin's got his prison teaching, of course, and just last week I was offered a full-time English teaching gig at a community college near the airport. The job starts in January, after the baby arrives, and it's tenure-track—which means it has the potential to be a forever-kind-of-job. Not that a forever-kind-of-job is something I'd normally get excited about, but hey. Making a baby doesn't leave room for our usual heady, middle-of-the-night decisions to quit everything, run off to some exotic country and work for peanuts. Now, it's about putting down roots, bringing in a steady stream of dough. At least that's what the world tells me, and I have no reason not to believe them.

"Putting down roots" must also mean, as I said before, buying a house. No suburban ramblers for us, thanks—this isn't our parents' day and age—but a house nonetheless. We fall in love instantly with the very first one we see: a small, old bungalow with a bright purple exterior, a big backyard bursting with pretty foliage, and a vintage RCA stove from the 1950s. And now that I've got some paychecks on the horizon, we can afford it, more or less. We put in an offer on the spot, and it is accepted a bit too quickly by the owner. This makes me briefly wish we'd offered less, but oh well.

To me, owning this small, purple house is of paramount importance, a central figure in our future parenthood fairytale. When I look at this house and the lush green rectangle of land around it, I don't just see a house with a yard. I see myself sitting contently on the deck with our new baby on my lap, watching Kevin rakes leaves, all of us bundled up in autumn-colored woolen clothing with our breath showing in the chilly air. I see Nina and David spontaneously appearing at the back gate to say hello— or maybe Bruce and Carrie or Jane and Jayson. I see Kevin setting down his gardening tools and pulling off the gloves, and all of us heading inside to hold each others' warm, new infants and talk about baby-oriented things like poop and booby milk. I see myself feeling warmly grateful to have such friendships.

And farther into the future, I see our child crawling on that linoleum kitchen floor, soon morphing into a bona fide person who can talk and think independently, saying only intelligent things because of the fish oil supplements that I'm dutifully consuming now. I see him or her lying on a bunk bed and flipping through comic books, walls decked out with posters of the latest child star. I see Kevin out in that yard again, teaching our child-formerly-known-as-baby how to hit a whifle ball with a red plastic bat, a second chance to do that. I hear the ball ricocheting loudly off the fence as the two of them chase and throw and catch, and Kevin saying, *Good! You got it!*, as I heat up lasagna in that vintage RCA oven.

By then, I will truly be in Nina's league of positive thinking, and ranking right up there with Carrie's seasoned and knowing calmness. I will have folded the trauma of my past into my soul, yet carried on with dignity and hope to create a new life. I'll be satisfied with everything I have, wanting nothing more, and Kevin will be pleased to have back the person that he married. I might even feel beautiful again, and we might even return to having regular sex.

All of these imaginary details are like life-puzzle pieces hovering around me, and it astounds me how easily I can throw them together inside my mind to create a complete picture. I refrain from sharing this splendid brain-candy with Kevin (who—if he did have a similar mental picture—would never admit it). Until this baby arrives safe and sound, I'll just be a lone reveler in the future—and I'm cool with that.

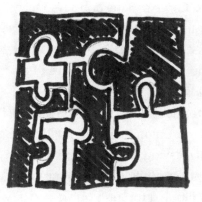

# A MYSTICAL CREATURE IN MY POCKET

IN THE END, PREGNANCY BOILS DOWN to a private, mother-child affair. Even as the belly grows to the point of being noticeable to others, the baby inside it is like some mystical forest creature that nobody but the mom knows exists, a little furry animal that she secretly keeps in her pocket and feeds sunflower seeds.

As spring turns into sun-drenched Seattle summer, I'm finally prego for real: belly-popping, double-chinning, boob-hurting, baby-name-researching, achingly-eager pregnant. Driving thirty minutes each way to my summer teaching job, acutely aware of transporting not just myself but a mini-someone else, I stay resolutely in the slow lane. No zipping past everyone at fifteen miles over the speed limit like I usually do; there's a baby on board! It's like that night-before-leaving-on-a-big-vacation feeling, when you're running around packing and watering your plants.

Jane sends out handmade invitations for my upcoming baby shower, and Mom calls every other day to check on my belly status while Dad listens in from the bedroom phone. Nina and Carrie and I get together for walks around Green Lake. We move like confident giraffes, slowly but proudly, holding our heads up high, talking animatedly about our tiredness and food cravings. Of course, there are still the prego group gatherings too, but I haven't much need for the other mommies-to-be anymore, now that I've got Nina and Carrie firmly in place as girlfriends.

Kevin has finally caught up with me on this blissful trajectory toward parenthood. His enthusiasm is more muted, channeled into practical matters: getting paternity leave forms signed, ensuring we have just the right amount of cash in just the right account, book-marking kid-friendly hotels overseas for our first trip. Still the military scout, he is extra-protective and aware of the space immediately surrounding my midsection, holding open doors and pulling me away if a table's corner or a counter's edge comes too near, controlling the things that he knows he can control. God help us both if I manage to screw this one up by tripping on a curb or running into something sharp.

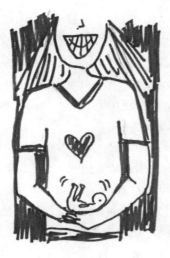

Still, even with all this community involvement in baby-growing, I often feel like the only one with a clear sense of our child's aliveness. I've been trying for the past few weeks to get Kevin to feel the baby "kick," if you could even call it kicking. It's more like a dull, rolling swoosh, and it only comes about once a day—sometimes twice if I'm lucky. Sometimes not at all. Day after day, hour after hour, I wait for those rare moments of movement. Usually, by the time Kevin rushes over to where I'm standing with my shirt yanked up, pointing to a precise spot on my round belly, he's missed it.

"Damn! I *just* felt it!"

"Next time," he says, not seeming to mind as much as I do.

I find it mildly bothersome that I'm the only one who ever really *feels* these sporadic swooshes, because if nobody else feels them, how will the world know that our little person is in there? It just seems sad to me that a baby's entire life in utero would go unfelt by others. So I keep at it, forcing Kevin to rest his hand on my stomach while we're reading on the sofa, hoping for some action at just the right time. And it's always the second he takes away his hand that the baby goes *swoosh*, not unlike that dancing cartoon frog who never performs when its owner wants him to.

Like I said: pregnancy is a mother-child affair.

## Sea of Explanations

ONE MIGHT THINK A MISCARRIAGE turns a woman into a nervous wreck the second time around. For me, it's had the opposite effect. That's because the idea of two pregnancies going wrong—one right after the other—has seemed so statistically, mathematically, and cosmically implausible that it's hardly been worth worrying about.

Until now, that is.

Here's the problem, and I realize this sounds like an utterly boring and common thing to be concerned about: *our baby isn't moving enough*. At least not as much as I would have hoped for, being nearly eight months along. I know, I know. That's, like, *the* most common concern among pregnant women who reach my big-bellied stage. And of course, it's usually okay, at least according to the books and websites eagerly throwing information in your face. But in my case, it's gotten to be more than just a bother, something I can make light of, like *such the perpetual sleepyhead!* or *our little night-owl must only be active while I'm asleep!*

Oh, there's the occasional lump of something pressing against my searching palm, or a soft flutter of motion from time to time. But whenever Carrie and Nina tell stories of frequent, whopping thuds against their insides, I look down pensively and rest my hands on my stomach, wondering with an unsettled feeling why I can't relate. Wishing I could see straight through my ribbed maternity tank top and taut skin, past the walls of my uterus and into my child's dark, watery, elusive world, just to check in.

Here's the aggravating part: when a baby doesn't move very much, there's always an explanation. A logical, medically sound explanation that any reasonable person would accept. I won't bother going into the details of those explanations. Just trust me, they're there: on the pages of *What to Expect When You're Expecting*, the universally accepted bible of purported pregnancy truth. On the tip of the nurse's tongue during one of my frequent evening calls. Kevin has them stored up too, those explanations, culled from Google. He busts them out at the pizza joint when I start feeling my tummy with one hand, balancing a cheese slice on the other, and staring distractedly off into space. Without having to ask, he knows what I'm worrying about. And boom: out comes an explanation. *Every baby moves differently. It depends on what you eat. As long as there's some movement, you're fine.*

If you don't accept these explanations, that must make you unreasonable. And who in the world wants to be unreasonable? Not me; that's for sure. So I reluctantly go along with them, suppressing the arc of panic when it rises inside my head, distracting myself with grading essays and perusing garage sale announcements for baby clothes.

ONE MORNING, I WAKE UP after a particularly restless night, bleary eyed and unable to stop yawning, and pour myself a half-cup of coffee to slurp on my drive to work. A wee bit of caffeine can't hurt anyone, can it? After my first few sips, I instantly feel more alert and chipper—better all around—and think wistfully back to the days when I could chug caffeine with unfettered, gluttonous bliss. Ah, those glorious hyper-productive mornings of regular and substantial bowel movements!

*See what I sacrifice for you?* I glance downward. *Hurry up and get here.* Eyes glued to the freeway, I set my travel mug on the armrest and rub my quiet tummy, hoping for a rare flutter. But as the morning progresses, I don't get the flutter I was hoping for. This time things seem even quieter than normal in there—no dull swooshes, not even a wisp of movement— and that familiar kernel of fear clamps around my heart. Soon, I'm standing before my students with words coming out of my mouth, my arm raised mechanically as I diagram sentences on the board. What I'm really thinking about is what's going on—or not going on—inside my belly.

"Um, I'm going to let you go a few minutes early today," I say, resting against the edge of my desk, my cheeks warm and flushed. "Don't forget we have a quiz tomorrow."

One of my students lingers after everyone has filed out of the room. It's Nancy, an older Puerto Rican woman with a gaggle of children of her own. "Ms. LeMoine, can I touch your stomach?"

"Sure. Go ahead."

She puts her hand right over my belly button, and leaves it there for several seconds.

"I don't feel him moving around in there, so he's probably sleeping. I think it's a boy, by the way. You ought to go home and get some rest. See you tomorrow, Ms. LeMoine."

"Okay. Bye Nancy."

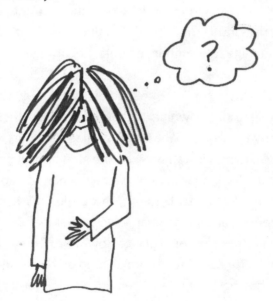

I walk back to my car and sit there behind the wheel for a moment before whipping out my cell phone. With shaky fingers, I dial the Group Heath consulting nurse for the third or fourth time this week. Her direct number is etched in my brain.

"Hi, this is Monica LeMo—"

"Oh yes, hello again. It's Carmelita. What's going on today, Monica?"

"Carmelita! Hi! Um, how do I say this? I think the baby might be dead." I pause for a moment to see if she reacts, but she doesn't. "I haven't felt any movement since last night, literally. I'm not kidding this time. Oh, and I drank like half a cup of coffee this morning, which I know probably wasn't the best idea, but—can I just come in to get checked out?"

"Sure, honey. Come on down. Drive carefully, now. And by the way—a cup of coffee's just fine."

Thirty minutes later, I'm lying down with sticky gelatinous stuff rubbed all over my abdomen, a different nurse hovering over me—this one I've never met before. She presses a gadget against my skin below the belly button and moves it in slow circles, not speaking. I watch her rings of brown hair flecked with silver, white squares of light reflected in her glasses, the fluorescent-lit ceiling panels above her. Breathing quietly on the edge of a cliff, waiting to be pushed off with her words: *I'm not finding anything.* A bulletin board covered with haphazardly thumbtacked pictures of newborns and thank you cards takes up a large part of the wall. *Thank you,* I envision them saying, *for doing your job. Please find the enclosed token photograph of my baby, because you don't get to see enough bald-headed, squinty-eyed babies around here.*

And then, rising out of the silence, the sound of an infant heartbeat emerges, rhythmic and unmistakable. *My infant,* the one underneath my belly skin. I swallow dryly, wishing I had a glass of water.

"Okay?" says the nurse, looking at my face. "Sounds completely normal and healthy."

"Mmm-kay," I say, though the spooked feeling still lingers. "But how come I hardly ever feel any movement?"

"Some babies just aren't as active as others."

See? A rational explanation, just as I expected. It should help, but it doesn't. Tears form before I can stop them, and one rolls out and down the side of my cheek. I wipe it away with the back of my palm, taking a deep and ragged breath, willing my lower lip to stop trembling. "Sorry. I'm just…I don't know. Scared."

"It's okay, honey. Like I said, every baby moves differently, and every mother feels differently. "

"Okay. Thanks." I feel better, I guess. I should feel better, anyway. She's a medical professional. I'm not. Driving home, biting down on the inside of my cheek, I push the fear back down like disgusting bile. Deep down, I know that living in fear is no way to live. Mom would tell me to enjoy these last eight weeks of pregnancy.

When I get home, I call Nina. "Wanna go get a pregnancy massage and go bikini shopping? Baby and I need to relax and feel sexy."

"Dude, totally. Let's do it! Best time to wear a two-piece is when you're preggers. Hides the belly flab."

Good old Nina-time. It's just what I need.

# MOTHER NATURE REARS HER HEAD

I'M LYING IN A DARKENED RADIOLOGY ROOM, green buttons glowing around me and medical equipment humming softly, my hair spread out on the pillow like a fan. Kevin is at home, probably awake by now and sitting at the kitchen table in his boxers, reading the *Seattle Times* sports section and sipping lukewarm coffee. I told him not to bother getting up early for this one even though he offered, because it's just a routine ultrasound—something they do at the seventh- or eighth-month mark. I've been feeling strangely unworried these past few weeks, my earlier bout of panic having mysteriously subsided. *Must just be a quiet baby*, I've come to casually accept. Thank goodness our brains can't simmer in heart-pumping anxiety mode forever; just imagine if they could! We'd all be running around like panicked freaks.

The radiologist is a balding, expressionless man who says nothing as he mechanically runs a wand over my KY Jelly-slathered belly. I keep my eyes on the round clock above the door.

"I'm just going to look this way, okay?" I say. "Just in case there's, like, an obvious penis or something showing up. We're trying not to know the gender. Anyway, how's he lookin' in general? Still alive, right?"

The minute hand shifts loudly. 9:24. Damn, I hope this dude hurries up. I've got twenty miles to drive and a stack of papers to copy before class starts. After a long pause, he says flatly, "Alive? Why do you ask?"

The fact that he doesn't immediately say "yes" doesn't go over my head, but I dismiss it. Clearly, he's trained to do radiology—not engage in small talk. He must not be married, nor have been around emotional

83

pregnant women who ask those questions specifically in order to get an enthusiastic, resounding, "Yes."

"Well, he—or she, whatever—has been kind of slow and sluggish lately." I shift my gaze to the rectangular ceiling panels above me, focusing on their shadowy cork-like surface as I blink my eyes, waiting.

"Yes, the fetus is still alive," he finally says, turning to leave the room. "I'm going to run these images back to show the head radiologist. Be right back."

Fetus?

Okay, call it what you will. Given my pro-choice voting record, I suppose I should be calling it a "fetus" too. The clock ticks audibly again; still time to get to class. I roll over onto my side, facing away from the screen with my head resting on my outstretched arm. The air feels good on my neck when my hair is pushed back—even this unmoving, KY-jelly-scented air. I close my eyes and shift my focus to the wondrous, intimate presence of two in the room. Not one, but two. As a rush of giddy motherliness hits me, I smile faintly in the darkness, feeling distinctly alive, human. I love these silent moments in a quiet examination room, when you're waiting for some doctor or nurse to show up. It's one of the best times to just chill in a Zen-like state, a perfect excuse to do nothing but relax.

Suddenly, the door bursts open, startling me out of my thoughts. It's the bald radiologist with a statuesque suit-clad woman striding in behind him.

"There's something wrong with your baby," she says in a vaguely European accent, pointing at the monitor. "We can see fluid and swelling throughout the body, between the organs. Run upstairs and see Dr. Williams right away—she already knows you're coming. Jim will show you to the stairs."

She turns on her heel and disappears, leaving me awkwardly alone with the bald radiologist, stunned speechless. I stare at him agape, this traitor who surely saw this coming. He averts his eyes, no doubt wondering anxiously how much time he has left before I lose my composure. One thing I've come to realize is that most men would rather eat dog turds than be sequestered in a room with a hysterical woman.

"I'll, uh, leave you alone to get dressed," he mutters and steps out into the hall.

In quick succession, random details flash inside of my head in red font: *fluid…swelling…organs.* Swelling? Like, swelling *up*? Like Augustus Gloop in *Charlie and the Chocolate Factory*? Is my kid about to burst? Will I have baby guts and amnio fluid streaming out of every orifice in my body, propelled by the sheer force of the explosion? And more important, *was it the coffee?*

There isn't much "getting dressed" to be done. I yank down my moss green maternity shirt—right over that residual film of KY Jelly on my skin—and impulsively unsnap my bra, sliding it through my sleeve (an old trick I learned in summer camp). Physical comfort is going to be key today if I'm expected to think straight, and that means freely swinging boobs. I wad it up and stuff it in my bag, right beside a stack of student essays. They'll never know their papers were snug up against their instructor's sweaty undergarment.

The radiologist leads me down the hallway and points to a darkened stairwell, saying nothing. Moving on auto-pilot, I climb up what feels like a never-ending series of flights, breathing hard, fumbling for my phone, dialing Kevin at home. Words tumble from my mouth: *something's wrong with the baby.* His voice is predictably calm as he asks what I know so far, and even calmer when I tell him the truth: not much, just general wrongness with the baby. He'll be right over, he says. With military precision, not overreacting until all facts are present. I find his words to be momentarily soothing, a cool and refreshing tendril of rationality. If this is one of those major life catastrophes that only happen to people on the Jerry Springer show, I would like to think I can handle it with grace and dignity. I suck air into my lungs, willing myself to stay calm, and pull open the heavy door at the top of the stairs.

A nurse appears immediately to usher me into Dr. Williams's office, where I'm told to wait. Left alone, I glance around at the framed photos on the shelves of Dr. Williams and her family. A husband, presumably. Two cute brown-haired boys—both teenagers, one taller than the other. Her sons. I wonder if she takes them for granted. A bus honks loudly on 15th Avenue outside, and nurses in the hallway behind me chat about faxing a chart. Not my chart; some other random person's chart. I guess that my own world's freezing to a halt doesn't mean the rest of reality does. Strange.

"Monica."

It's Dr. Williams in the doorway, her eyes crinkly and kind as she extends her arms and encloses me in a hug. She feels thin beneath her white lab coat, shoulder blades pointy, long brown-and-silver hair smelling vaguely like flowery shampoo. I feel hollow and buzzing inside, like a carved out tree trunk full of bumblebees, and I pull away.

"Well?" I say.

The million-dollar question. Before she opens her mouth to speak, I already know the answer, just from the way her dark eyebrows furrow a tiny bit. She's going to tell me that the radiologist was right. It's bad. Holy-fucking, bitch-smacking bad. I chomp on the inside of my cheek and send a mental note to Mother Nature: bring it on, bee-yatch. This is one fight I don't plan on losing.

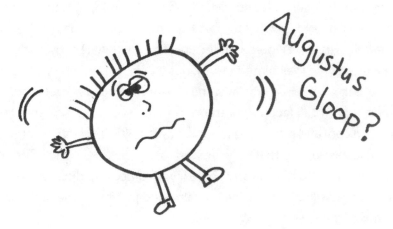

## To Feel Like a Family

KEVIN AND I ARE SITTING on a floral patterned sofa in a corner room at the University of Washington Medical Center, fingers laced together hard. I keep noticing how handsome he looks with his jaw set, face unshaven, eyes slightly narrowed like they always are when he's in serious concentration mode. He does it during Scrabble games, too. Not that this is the time or place to be thinking about such things. *God, we're up a shit's creek.*

Before us is a row of grave-faced doctors in lab coats, clipboards in their arms. Dr. Lee, a tall dark-haired woman with thin-rimmed glasses, does the talking.

"Monica, Kevin, your baby is dying from massive heart failure. The heart failure has led to hydrops—fluid-back up and swelling from head to feet to scrotum. I'm very sorry. There isn't anything we can do."

*Scrotum.* I heard that. Didn't I tell them we're keeping the gender a secret? I blink several times and look at Kevin. We're losing this fight after all, puzzle pieces flying apart. I feel small inside.

"You're certain?" he says, voice low. Just getting the facts straight before jumping to conclusions. Good tactic.

"Yes."

"There's nothing that can be done?" he says. "No treatment?"

"No. I'm sorry."

He breathes in deeply and exhales, still looking forward, and slowly nods as pain registers on his face. Meanwhile, an odd and unexpected sensation of foul-tasting relief settles into my system. Relief about having some certainty: a definitive—albeit horrific—prognosis. At least there aren't any false hopes, no experimental new surgical procedures that probably won't work (but might), no flying a preemie-sized heart over from a sketchy Pakistani organ dealer that probably won't do any good (but might). Just a solid rung of unquestionable information to hang onto: *nothing can be done.*

"You have several options," Dr. Lee continues. That's what I like to hear: options. Let's see what tricks this smart lady has up her sleeve. "You could continue to carry the pregnancy, and allow him to pass away on his own. This could take hours or days, possibly even a full month or more. We just don't know."

Kevin and I look at each other, than back at her. Keep being pregnant with a baby who's dying but not totally dead? Not conducive to getting on with life. Certainly a recipe for a nervous breakdown, or an identity crisis, or both.

"What else is there?" I say.

"We could induce labor now, although his survival for any length of time outside the uterus is unlikely. He wouldn't be in good shape when he came out. We would give him pain medicines, wrap him in a blanket, and hand him over to you."

"Hand him over to *us?* What for? I mean, what could we do for him?"

"Say goodbye."

This sounds so terrifying that I can hardly stomach the thought of it. I don't know how to hold my infant son and wait for him to die. That's not something anyone ever taught me, not in high school, or even college. Kevin's eyes are glistening in the natural light coming in through the window, and he grabs a tissue from the bedside table and gently blows his nose. Horror grips my insides, but I shove it down and try to concentrate.

"The third option would be to terminate and deliver him stillborn," Dr. Lee says. "That would be a painless procedure involving an injection to the baby's heart. You and the baby wouldn't feel a thing."

Terminate. *Wouldn't feel a thing.*

The words hover before me in the air, light and feathery, safe-sounding. Almost magical.

"We'll leave you two alone to discuss." They all shuffle out of the room with their heads down, the last one shutting the door behind him. Kevin tilts his head back against the edge of the sofa, staring at the ceiling.

"What do you think?" he says softly.

"I don't know. What do you think?"

"I asked you first."

"Fine, be that way. Force your poor wife to talk first on the most depressing day of her life."

"I think we need to do what's most humane for the baby and for us."

He turns toward me and lowers his head, slipping his hand beneath my aqua green gown to caress my enormous belly underneath. Just then, I feel a flutter inside. A small protruding bump moves slowly across my taut skin.

"I felt that," he murmurs. I nod my head, stroking his sideburns and the edge of his baseball cap, growing intensely conscious of there being three of us now. Three of us, perhaps for the last time: a family. It's the only way we can be a family of sorts, with Kevin feeling the aliveness of his child—this little unseen person with a scrotum. *A boy.*

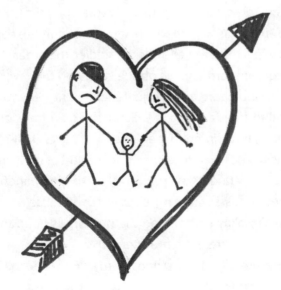

I look down at my belly, and something forces a sob up from deep within me. It's got nothing to do with putting together any pieces of life, covering any bases, or getting anywhere at all. It's just an ice-cold, crystal clear feeling slicing through my torso, achingly and humanly real. Knowing, hurting more than anything has ever hurt: *I'm going to lose you.*

GETTING A GRIM PROGNOSIS is so bewildering compared to how I always imagined it would be, so anti-climactic. It was like this in Arkansas, too. No single soap-opera note in minor key, no promise of a perky commercial jingle to lighten the mood, no accompanying instruction manual on what to think or feel or say. Sure, you've got doctors dishing out facts and numbers—but nobody offers up any simple formulas for consuming those facts, digesting them. The bad news just gets dropped on top of your head like a big, confusing shit sundae: BOO-YA. And guess who gets to deal with the mess? Not your mom, not your friends, not God, not your teacher, not your maid, not your dog. Nope; it's all you. You, you, you.

Or in this case, it's Kevin and me. We hold one another up like puppets, taking turns attending to real-world practical matters. Time feels slow and syrupy as we propel ourselves through the day. While one of us stares into space like a shell-shocked soldier, the other chats with the nurses, signs consent forms, fields phone calls. And then we switch.

Each increasingly rare and languid movement beneath my tummy skin is like a mind trick: a dying, swollen baby now transforming into a mysterious entity, hovering between dead and alive. He feels as though he's already mostly gone, transformed into a cloud of baby dust, blowing elusively through my fingers as I frantically try to grab handfuls of it. And with his realness goes something else: my own sense of being a real, feeling person. I'm okay with letting the numbness flood in like a tepid sea of gray, for now. Better than the alternative.

Kevin helps me adjust the strings of my frumpy hospital gown. My heart is beating louder than normal against my chest, but there's no reason to be nervous, I tell myself. At least I know what's coming. He turns me around and puts his hands on my shoulders, looking directly down into my eyes. The past few hours, he's seemed sad and stoic in a guy-ish way, while monitoring me from under the rim of his baseball cap.

"Are you gonna be alright?" he says.

"Yeah. It's weird, but I feel pretty much fine." Numb, I want to say, but "fine" sounds better. "Let's just get this over with."

A nurse leads us into a small room full of machines. I lie down and stare up at the fluorescent-lit ceiling panels above, and Kevin sits beside me, holding my hand, watching me intently. A group of doctors assembles around us, talking in low voices to one another, mostly clinical terminology that I don't understand. Dr. Lee is also there, and I find her presence soothingly familiar.

There's a brief flutter of movement in my abdomen, what I can only imagine to be a few painful, final arm and leg stretches. I clutch Kevin's hand and shut my eyes. As the doctors turn on machines and the lights grow dim, I feel suddenly filled with terror, like a criminal awaiting execution. They're not killing *me*, I remind myself; just a *piece of me*. Still, panic jars me inside, and like a frightened animal I start to pant and shake. Kevin holds onto my arm, whispering *relax*. His warm skin and voice make me feel grounded in something earthly and normal.

"So, Monica," says Dr. Lee, her voice quiet and gentle. "We're going to insert chemicals into the fetal heart with a long needle. We'll be using an ultrasound picture to guide us. Everyone here is very experienced, so you're in good hands. You and the baby won't feel a thing. It's just going to stop his heart, okay?"

"'Kay."

Someone rubs cool, sticky stuff all over my tummy and turns on a machine. I feel a little bit better.

"Would you like some anti-anxiety meds, honey?" asks a nurse. "Something just to numb the brain for a while?"

"Ummmmm…" I hesitate, just because I still think anti-anxiety meds sound like something for crazy people, but then I remember that sometimes numbness is a lifesaver. "Sure."

The drug swiftly goes into me through an IV needle, its effects instantaneous, coating my mind in a warm fog of blissful delirium. It's like I'm here but not really, babbling nonsensically to Kevin that the TV in the corner looks upside down, and that my right toe itches like crazy, and that a Frappucino from Starbucks would sure taste good right now. I can hear my voice, feel my lips moving, but my mind is miles away. And before I know it, it is over.

The only reason I know it's over is that I've somehow ended up in the room where we started, where people are lifting me into bed like I'm some kind of invalid. Kevin is next to me, talking softly to a nurse. Through the rainbow fog of my mind, I have a fleeting picture of my baby's soul up above, jumping up and down and applauding wildly now that the pain, the swollenness, is finished. That's fine and all; I'm happy for him. But what's really making me smile in barely perceptible, Mona-Lisa-sort-of way—aside from the happy drugs—is that even though that chapter of my life is officially dead, Kevin and I are still alive.

Only one more big hurdle to go.

# THE FINAL PUSH

WE'RE IN THE HOMESTRETCH: once again holed up in a hospital room, jacked up on labor-inducing pills, and left to wait. A return to that exotic parallel universe of last summer, the one where people look pregnant but really aren't, and where women expel large, inanimate objects from their vaginas. I wonder if I'll violently vomit and shit, too, completing the full déjà vu experience.

Kevin and I attempt to laugh about normal things. We analyze the hospital menu, discussing things like what "Salisbury steak" really is, and flip through the TV channels for laugh-worthy infomercials. I avoid touching my protruding belly, for fear of recognizing the shape of a little lifeless foot or elbow pressed against my insides. That would surely make me sadder than I know how to be, rendering me incapable of the formidable task of delivering this baby, which I hope to do today. Baby corpse, I mean. Christ. Kevin doesn't touch my belly, either—and the nurses swarming in and out hardly give it a second glance. It's like the invisible elephant that nobody wants to talk about.

A social worker named Joanne shows up with a clipboard and a stack of papers. She's wearing a fuzzy, peach-colored sweater and looks about twenty years older than me. Deep down, I'm glad Joanne is here. Perhaps she was sent by society at large to guide us with profoundly useful and comforting information.

"How are you two feeling?" she asks, peering above the rim of her glasses.

"Fine," Kevin and I say in unison. She frowns and jots something down on her clipboard, handing us some glossy pamphlets. The top one is called

93

"Stages of Grief." I wonder if—once again—we are fucking everything up, giving the wrong answers, not following the stages in order.

"The doctor tells me you don't have plans to hold the baby," she says. "You should really think about holding him for a while once he's born, calling him by name. Research shows this is the best thing to do."

"Um, probably not, but we'll think about it." My eyes flicker to Kevin, who is nodding in what I hope is silent agreement. I have yet to hear a single convincing argument in favor of holding one's own dead infant.

Sometime in the wee hours of the night, I begin to feel as though a metal vice is clamping down on my ovaries. A pair of mousy, young nurses arrives, sticking an epidural needle into my backside and pulling my feet up into stirrups.

"It's time to push," one of them says, and I take their word for it. Kevin stands beside me and holds my hand. I close my eyes and bear down as hard as I can, becoming inexplicably hot and thirsty.

"He's moving pretty slow," somebody says. "Just keep pushing."

I breathe for a moment and then try again, this time for what seems like hours. I can hear the nurses sighing and shuffling and whispering to one another. Why doesn't someone tell me something useful besides just "push?" Pushing obviously isn't working. As piercing cramps course through my abdomen, I become even hotter and thirstier than before, and start to violently shake and sweat. Nobody told me it would be this…*hard*. And sorry, but whoever said the epidural shot actually makes childbirth a pain-free experience is full of shit. I'm sure the nurses are wondering what to do with this incapable, trembling woman who obviously never bothered to take childbirth classes. Perhaps they didn't get the memo that it's a *dead* baby I'm trying to expel, not a *real* baby, and that therefore I ought to be given some baby-delivery Cliff's Notes, a few short cuts.

"I can't do this," I finally say through chattering teeth, letting my knees fall together as my head falls back on my pillow. Screw it; I'm taking a nap, whether these people like it or not. It feels as though I have an enormous rugby ball lodged halfway inside me, but I'm too tired and feverish to care. There's a flurry of activity near my feet, the door opening and closing.

Kevin's hand remains planted on mine, and within moments I've slipped into a half-sleeping state. Just as I begin to dream, a new doctor with an unfamiliar voice comes bursting through the door, elbowing past the others in the room.

"Okay, Monica, you can do this," she says, her voice booming, oozing confidence and certainty. "You're going to do exactly as I say, and you're going to deliver this baby. Work now, sleep later. Let's do it!"

"Mmmm?" I raise my eyelids halfway to get a better look at this military commando woman ordering me around. She's pretty and young, with brown hair pulled back in a ponytail and a shower-cap-looking thing on her head. Her voice is low and teacher-ish like Nina's, and I instantly feel compelled to impress her with my baby-expelling finesse. "Arright," I mumble. For her.

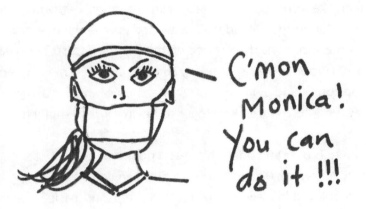

I concentrate on the dimly lit ceiling as she talks to me in a combination cheerleader/swim instructor voice, loudly telling me exactly what to do and when. *Inhale. Hold it. Now push for ten seconds. Super! Exhale for five. Inhale. Hold it. Excellent! You're almost there! Push for ten seconds. You're doing great, Monica!* Being bossed around by a pretty doctor with a low voice really isn't half bad. In fact, I'm sort of getting into it, imagining disco music playing in the background. And within minutes, the baby comes out with a *whoosh* sensation, and I am instantly flooded with the most physically euphoric, exhausted feeling ever.

The room is as quiet as my son's body, which gets immediately whisked away by the mousy, whispering nurses. Someone mentions *tear, stitches*…but I figure it's best not to know what they're talking about. As Kevin says something tender into my ear, I fall instantly to sleep. Soon I'm dreaming about adopting that pretty, brown-haired military doctor who just saved my life, taking her home so she can be my personal life coach forever. I think I might even have a crush on her.

WHEN I WAKE UP, IT'S NEARLY EIGHT in the morning, and rays of sunlight are slanting into our room. Kevin is sound asleep on the sofa, and a tray of scrambled eggs has been placed in front of me. My entire crotch feels like somebody assaulted it with a baseball bat, but other than that, I feel gloriously fine and well rested, relieved—again—to be alive. An enormous weight has been lifted off my mind and torso, now that our epic tale of corpse-delivery has finally come to an end. Time to get out of this frumpy outfit and get home, take a real shower and check my e-mail.

"Hey, time to get up," I call over to Kevin. "Rise-n-shine! It's coffee time!"

As he rolls over and opens his eyes, I pour two packets of sugar into the watery, lukewarm Maxwell House accompanying my breakfast, down it in three quick gulps, and hit my red "Call" button to ask for a second cup.

Within seconds, there's a gentle knock on the door, and I shout "Come in!", marveling at how fast the coffee-delivery service is around here. It's a blond nurse with crinkles of kindness in the corners of her eyes. She doesn't have any coffee.

"Hi Monica. I'm Doreen. I was there in the delivery room with you last night, but you probably don't remember. How ya doing this morning?"

"I'm feeling really good, actually. Just glad it's all over. What time do we get to go home?"

"I'll check with the doctor on that. I wanted you to know that you have a beautiful son. Everyone's talking about how remarkably cute he is, especially that nose. Where did he get that nose!"

Instantly, my mood dips down. Oh yeah—there's that. That's what last night's pushing and breathing and sweating was all about. I'd almost forgotten.

"His nose? I'm not sure where he got it." I look at her for a moment longer. "What makes you say that? I mean, what's his nose look like?"

"Well, we've given him a bath and taken some pictures of him for you to keep, so you can see for yourself. Actually, would you like me to bring him in so you can hold him?"

I turn my eyes toward Kevin, who is looking back at me. I'd really rather not, but it's hard to say no when you're put on the spot like this. Besides, if we don't do this, Doreen might run over and tell that social worker lady with the peach sweater, and she'd make a note of it on our permanent grieving record.

"Is he...like...wrapped in a blanket or anything?" Kevin asks.

"Yes, he's all swaddled up with his face covered," says Doreen.

"Well, okay," I say after a long pause, still looking at Kevin. "Okay, Kev?"

"Okay," he says.

"But just for a few minutes," I add, feeling as though I'm about to leap into the great, frightening unknown. Going to Uzbekistan for two-and-a-half years was nothing compared to this. Kevin sidles up next to me on the bed, and Doreen returns with an infant-sized thing in a light blue blanket, placing the bundle gently in my arms. She then ducks quietly out the door.

This is one of those situations in life where time stands still. I know that sounds cheesy, but it's true. I recognize that it's an important and real moment, and I try to concentrate on soaking it up. *Be here, in the present,* my brain tells me. *Be here, because you won't have this chance again.*

I clutch the silent object awkwardly against my chest, unsure of how to think about it, what to call it, how to categorize it in my mind. So this is the entity that's been growing inside me for nearly eight months, the blossoming seed of a child I've grown attached to, eaten for, slept for, avoided coffee for, dreamed about, imagined, anticipated. It's surprisingly heavy, this limp jumble of arms and legs with a little round head that I instinctively cradle with the palm of my hand.

When I lift the bundle upward so that part of it rests in the crook of my neck, it feels the way a real baby would feel. I breathe in to see what it smells like: baby soap. Baby powder. Kevin and I don't talk at all; we just take deep breaths and pass the bundle gingerly back and forth, clutching him against our bodies, being careful not to drop him.

"Let's see what he looks like," I hear myself say. I pull back a corner of the blanket with a trembling hand, and look down to see a tiny rosebud mouth, frozen open wide in what I can only imagine is an *oh shit!* exclamation of dismay. Kevin and I breathe in sharply at the same time, and I rush to cover it back up, stifling a deep and primal sob. It's more than I can bear. I feel massively duped, in fact, for almost falling for it. Foolish believing for a single second that this morbid, baby-like thing might, *just might,* turn into my living, breathing child if I pulled back that blanket and wanted it desperately enough. It worked (sort of) for Chuckie's dad, didn't it?

"I'm done when you are," says Kevin.

"Me too. Let's get outta here." I press the red call button and someone other than Doreen appears almost instantly, carrying my requested cup of coffee.

"Here, I'll trade you," I say without explanation, handing the blue bundle over to the confused-looking woman after she sets down my steaming Styrofoam cup. I must have a frightening look on my face, for she hurries out the room without saying a word. Won't she be shocked when she gets back out in the hallway and discovers she's got a dead baby in her arms. Just my own little way of ending this segment of my life with a dose of twisted humor, of getting back at whoever's controlling the gears up there for messing with my head. Maybe not so graceful, but it's all I can think to do.

# The Third Journey Segment:
## Detour Into a Bizarre, Snot-Laden Acid Trip
*August to October, 2007*

# Post-Dead-Baby Honeymoon Phase

NOBODY EVER TOLD ME THAT HAVING A BABY hurts like hell, not just during, but *after*. Physical, back-aching, vagina-stretching hell. Don't get me wrong; I'm not complaining. In fact, it's something I feel tremendously glad about at the moment. Let me explain.

Kevin and I arrive home from our extended hospital stay, dazed and baby-less. My vagina has, in fact, been stretched to eye-popping proportions. Aside from the flowers, cards, and casseroles left on the back porch, the house is devoid of evidence that I was ever pregnant at all. Jane and Jayson graciously came through earlier to tidy up the kitchen, gather up all of the baby books and infant outfits and other paraphernalia, and transfer them to the garage. Which is just as well, for I don't see any point in surrounding ourselves with all those un-puked-on blankies, un-pooped-in onesies, and un-slept-in bassinet. Unhelpful, depressing props. The *What to Expect* book has vanished too; it's as though nearly eight months of expectation have simply evaporated.

We do have a few concrete relics that the hospital sent us home with, and we empty them from our backpacks onto the bed. A blue satin "memory box," a clump of the baby's black hair, several sets of his tiny ink footprints on parchment paper, a handful of black and white photographs of his feet and profile, an official-looking certificate of birth and death for someone named Baby Boy LeMoine. They're like gameshow consolation prizes, and I'm not sure what to do with them. Display them on the fireplace mantel to collect dust? Kevin and I hold them up to the light together, examining them, trying to feel something from them.

Nothing.

There has to be *something*, though, and here's where the stretched-out vagina comes in. When the defining center of your life goes away, something else rises up like a volcano to take its place. For me, that most-welcomed volcano is the least savory souvenir of all: my bruised and sore post-partum body, and the task of caring for it. It's a task that requires a tremendous amount of energy and focus, leaving less focus for the terrible, aching silence of our purple bungalow house.

Take the something-degree tear in my perineum, for example. And if you're not sure what that is, go look it up right now; everyone should have "perineum" in their repertoire of impressive four-syllable vocabulary words to toss out at cocktail parties. I also have a newly blossoming hemorrhoid that feels like a hornet burrowing into my arse (and I know you know what a hemorrhoid is). As a result of these two ailments, or perhaps in addition to them, I've got elephantitis-like swelling of that whole general area between the legs. Which means I'm hobbling bow-legged around the house like an elderly woman who just had prolonged intercourse with a well-hung young man.

Nursing my body is a project that keeps me—and Kevin—mercifully busy, day after day. To keep the region cool and relatively unswollen, I store plastic baggies filled with ice cubes down my underwear (and you can bet it's granny-Hanes from here on out, as this weary body won't be partaking in scintillating foreplay anytime soon). As the ice begins to melt every twenty minutes or so, the bags inevitably leak in the corners, sending cold rivulets of water down my inner thighs. Sometimes I get so tired of changing out of wet clothes that I lie there in bed in a pool of frigid water, hoping it will just evaporate on its own. It never does.

There is still blood coming out of me—lots of it—which makes me wonder if my stitches are healing properly. My personal theory, which I explain to Kevin every night after he shuts off the bedside lamp, is that the stitches came partially undone while I was pooping, which means that poop molecules could very well be getting up in through the wound and into my blood stream, spreading infectious waste throughout my circulatory system. I ask him to feel my forehead every few hours, which he dutifully does and tells me I'm fine. I eventually fall asleep but only after twenty or thirty minutes of lying awake with my thoughts racing.

But the most time-consuming task of all, requiring more careful planning and concentration than any other part of my day, is the unavoidable act of pooping. I attack this challenge with determination, announcing loudly to Kevin each time: "I'M GOING TO THE BATHROOM! WISH ME WELL!"—as though I'm about to embark on a treacherous journey.

First, I clean the entire area with a Tucks medicated pad, one of my new favorite all-purpose cleaning-and-medicating products. Second, I gingerly release my bodily waste, being careful not to bear down too forcefully in the process, lest I pop my stitches open and spread infection, which I'm worried may have happened already. Third, I wipe from front to back with toilet paper, being ever so careful not to accidentally touch my stitches, which sting like needle pricks whenever they come in contact with anything. Fourth, I stand up and place a round plastic bin filled with warm water over the toilet seat and sit directly in it, so that my swollen and now-burning private parts are fully submerged. This is by far the most soothing part of my bathroom routine. I often just sit there for a while with my head resting in my hands, reflecting on the meaning of life, or skimming the outdated Target catalog still wedged in the magazine holder.

Eventually, Kevin notices the silence and asks through the door if I'm okay, and I tell him I'm fine. I like it when he frets over me like this, and wonder if he thinks I might have overdosed on Tylenol and drowned myself in the tub. After I've soaked to my own satisfaction, I grab a bar of Dial soap from the shower and gently cleanse the entire pooping-peeing region, rinsing with fresh water from a plastic cup. Another quick swipe of the whole area with a Tucks pad, a fresh coat of Preparation H, and a layer of numbing gel—all of which were provided to me in that nifty little consolation package from the hospital.

All the while, Kevin zips around like a star employee, tending to life's everyday chores: the grocery shopping, cooking, cleaning, refreezing and replacing my ice packs, running to the video rental store and back, taking phone calls. Picking up the slack because I'm beached on the futon like an invalid whale. It suits him, just like being beached suits me.

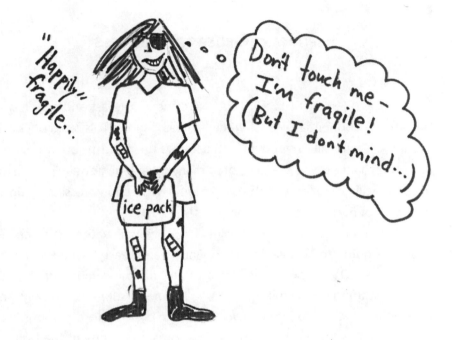

SEE? NOW YOU UNDERSTAND WHY the physical aftermath isn't so bad—more like a post-dead-baby honeymoon. What would Kevin and I do without this distraction-high? Here's what: we would both be forced to look squarely at our lives, at the stinging reality of the road behind and before us. That's where. I'll take a few physical challenges over that any day.

## Important Orders of Business

MY CROTCH-STITCHES ARE HEALING obnoxiously fast, and pooping is becoming exponentially easier with each passing day. This rapid physical healing is leaving all kinds of unwanted free space inside my brain. But not to worry! Thanks to the presence of so many other logistic details of life to tend to, I still get to fend off the black, liquid depression pressing against the doors of my psyche, threatening to seep in.

One important order of business is deciding whether to cancel what was going to be called the "Pre-Baby Dance Party" scheduled in a month or so. Don't ask me why I'm stuck on the dance party; it should be the last thing on my mind. The thing is, I'm not sure if technically I'm allowed to have any fun right now. What's the protocol for situations like this? Should Kevin and I be sequestering ourselves alone in the house, covering our faces and wailing in misery for months to come? Should my eyes be permanently puffy and red-rimmed? Will people see me having a good time and get suspicious of me for not appearing upset enough? God forbid someone think that I purposely gave my baby heart failure by ingesting that half-cup of coffee.

"What do you think about the dance party?" I ask Kevin, sidling up next to him in the living room. He's sitting on the futon with the phone in his lap, having just hung up with his mother.

"Dance party? What dance party?" Clearly, his mind is in other places.

"You know, the huge pre-baby bash we had going on next month, the one we already bought all that vodka for. Do you think it's still kosher to have a party at a time like this?"

Kevin looks over at me. "Screw what's kosher. Let's have the dance party." The millionth reminder of why my husband kicks ass. So it's decided: the dance party will stand. We're not going to let this colossal face-smack from Mother Nature ruin what was going to be a booty-shake fest in the basement.

Next logistical matter in line: my job. I was hired to start in January, which would have given me plenty of cushioning time to be home with the baby. Now, it suddenly seems hugely important that I start in the fall quarter instead, even though that's just a few weeks from now. If I wait until January, that means four-and-a-half months of being neither the new mommy I thought I would be, nor the career-driven, tenure-track instructor I've worked so hard to become. Meaning four-and-a-half months of being a direction-less nobody. Yuck.

"I guess I should tell Highline I can start right away," I say to Kevin as he's slathering peanut butter on a piece of flatbread.

"Are you sure you'll be ready? The quarter starts in…like three or four weeks, right?"

"Yeah, that's plenty of time to get over this whole thing."

Kevin looks up at me for a few seconds. "Might be good to start work, actually, just to give you something to focus on. Why don't you e-mail and see what they say?"

I go into the pastel yellow Office-Formerly-Known-as-Baby's Room, flip open the laptop, and hammer out a quick e-mail message to the department coordinator.

*8/23/07*

*Hi Winona, I hope you are doing well and enjoying your summer. The baby didn't work out, and I was wondering if it would be possible to begin full-time this September for fall quarter. Kevin and I both feel that getting on with our professional lives will really help us with the grieving and recovery process. The time when I feel best and strongest right now is when I'm busy and focused on other things that I really enjoy, such as teaching.*

Okay, so I pulled that last line out of my ass. I have no idea when I feel "best and strongest," since I haven't had time to do anything other than feel sore and numb. Still, it has a nice ring to it. I read my message several times, making sure that I come across as sufficiently level-headed and professional, lest Winona get the impression that I'm making any rash decisions about my readiness to teach. Satisfied, I hit "send."

I hope it's not too late, that they can fit me in the schedule, that they don't have some policy against bringing emotionally damaged instructors on board. In fact, I can hardly bear the thought of Winona saying no. I get up for a drink of water, pausing before the kitchen sink to imagine myself standing up before a class of sleepy college freshmen, resuming teaching as though a dead baby didn't just come out of my vagina. Heck, I've done it before, so why not do it again? My e-mail in-box is still showing when I return, and I click "refresh" to see if Winona happened to write back in the three minutes that I was gone. She didn't, and this gives me a twinge of anxiety.

But I try to think of what Kevin would say. He would tell me not to worry about things I can't control, like the date and time that Winona responds to my message. What's more, I've got lots more to look forward to: several whole weeks left of summer vacation with Kevin all to myself, not to mention all the visitors who keep arriving at our doorstep.

Winona writes back an excruciating twenty-four hours later, asking if I'm sure I'm ready for this. It's intense, she warns me. I tell her I'm fine, of course, sealing the deal: I am to report to work in a few short weeks. It's a relief to know that life goes on, even when there is death.

## Me Versus Mammary Glands

"GAAAHHH!"

Kevin jerks his head over toward me, suddenly awake. The digital clock shows 3:27 in the morning. "What is it?!"

"Something fucked up is happening! Look!"

I scramble over his body to flip on the lamp switch, and then—with both index fingers—point to two wet splotches on my t-shirt, right over my nipples. Kevin leans over and takes a close look at my chest, squinting in the lamp light, and then sighs and rolls back over on his side.

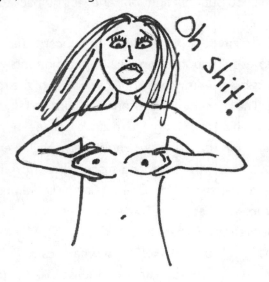

"Didn't the nurse say your body would start to, um, make milk?" he says, his voice scratchy from slumber.

Now that he mentions it, I do vaguely recall some nurse's voice coming through the leftover drug-induced haze the day we left the hospital, warning me this would happen. Wear two sports bras to compress the chest, she said, and stuff them with frozen peas and yogurt—or was it lima beans and cottage cheese? I remember briefly wondering how anyone had ever come up with this idea of turning one's chest into a legume-dairy casserole for the purpose of suppressing unwanted milk—was it a serendipitous finding that started out as some strange sexual fetish? *Darling...go dig up something cool from the fridge, and rub it all over my chest!* It didn't matter anyway, I thought, because my boobs would never do something so stupid as to switch into dairy mode at this inopportune time. No, no. *My* breasts would intuitively understand the circumstances, and know what not to do. So I thought.

"But...gawd!" I cry out. "Look how big and swollen and nasty they are!"

"Why don't you put on a tight bra, and let's go back to sleep. It's not even light out yet."

But by now, I'm so wide awake with concern that I may as well officially get up, even though it's only 3:27 in the morning (well, 3:28 now). So I pull a sports bra over my chest, quietly slip out of the room, and start a pot of coffee. The laptop is still on from last night, so I sit down before it, trying to decide what I can Google to make myself feel better.

"*Breast milk for sale,*" I type impulsively. Hell. Perhaps I could pump mine out, bottle the stuff, and make a bit of profit from all this horribleness—maybe even offer different flavors by adding chocolate or strawberry syrup. Not that I'd ever order some other woman's breast milk (ewww!) but someone out there might.

There isn't much of a market, from what I can tell. I come across an organization where you donate your breast milk for the children of "women less fortunate," but I skip past that one, because I'm not exactly in a charitable kind of mood. Shouldn't people be donating stuff to me? Sanity? Live babies? Cash? *I'm* the "less fortunate" one, dammit. There's also one anonymous person selling plastic bags of frozen "human breast milk" on Craigslist, with no price or location listed, which I find rather suspicious. Now that I think about it, doesn't it seem the slightest bit eerie to preface "breast milk" with the word "human" anyway? Isn't "breast milk" generally assumed to be from a human? And if not, how else could it be interpreted? Chicken breast milk? I doubt it.

The whole industry sounds sketchy. Quite possibly illegal, even. I picture the breast-milk-trafficking police knocking on my door with a warrant to search my house. I would have to frantically shove all my pumps and bottles under the mattress, while nervously shouting, "COME IN!!!" And if they got anywhere close to finding my incriminating paraphernalia, I'd have to resort to violence, squirting each officer in the face with a fast, hard stream of milk from each nipple.

As this image surfaces, my entrepreneurial spirit fizzles. It instead becomes my personal crusade to stop the milk onslaught at all costs, rather than try to be my own cash cow. And I'd better act fast, because once the milk-flow starts, it will become like a permanently leaky faucet in the basement, and I'll have to pump the stuff out until I'm fifty-something, my boobs becoming dried-up melons glued to my chest. At least, I've heard that's how it happens with dairy cows.

I begin wearing three sports bras at all times, obsessively pressing my palms against my chest to create a wall of force against the immense tidal wave of milk that I imagine to be just behind those nipples. It becomes a competition of sorts: me against the mammary glands. I stuff my not-so-secret weapons down my bras: plastic bags full of ice cubes and peas and spoonfuls of yogurt. I practice psychological warfare, too, glaring downward at my swollen breasts and willing the milk not to come. My battle against the boobs becomes the centerpiece of all conversations, with everyone rooting for me in what's now known as the "milk thing:"

"Hi honey, it's mom. How's the milk thing going?"

"Oh, fine. I think I'm winning out."

"Good for you. Keep me posted."

Or: "Hey, it's Jane. Everything okay with the milk thing?"

"Yeah, I just replaced my ice pack. I think I'm in the lead."

IN THE END, EXCEPT FOR A FEW TRACES that leak out and leave little yellowish rings on my bra, I end up defeating my boobs in a stunning victory. Somehow, though, it isn't a victory that I feel particularly good about.

"Looks like I won," I tell Kevin halfheartedly, braless for the first time in a week. "I think my boobs are shrinking back to normal size. Maybe we can like...have sex soon." The thought of sex makes me inwardly cringe, but Kevin might appreciate a token mention of the act.

"Good."

"Yeah," I say, tightness rising in my stomach. Tears prick at my eyeballs, and I blink them back. "Good, I guess."

# MAKING UP RULES

WEDDINGS AND LIVE-BABY BIRTHS are easy. The world is perfectly set up to handle them, and everyone knows exactly what to do. There are zillions of cards and invitations designed specfically to announce that this person is marrying that person, or baby-blah-blah was born. There are clear-cut, template ways to behave and converse about such things, and a preapproved set of gifts that are socially appropriate to give and receive. Even funerals aren't anything new; they happen everyday, on TV, in real life. We know what they are; we understand them.

Stillbirth, on the other hand, is unchartered territory for everyone—especially for the "parents" like us—if you could call us "parents." It starts with the very basic question of what to call the baby. Without ever really talking about it, we've somehow settled on just that: "the baby." And because there aren't any formal rules of etiquette stating whether a stillborn baby should be called "the baby" or "the fetus" or something else entirely, we're left to act according to our instinct-of-the-day.

Months ago, we picked out a girl-name and a boy-name: Anna and Zachary. These seemed perfect; that much we hardly debated. I still can't imagine there being anywhere on earth two more suitable names for a LeMoine child. We never told anyone about the boy-name, and neither of us dares to utter it now. It somehow seems unnatural to me, even a bit tacky, to suddenly start referring to our lost infant as "Zachary." It's not as though we ever called him "Zachary" before. Hell, we didn't even know it was a boy. Who are we to now pretend we knew him all along, his name and gender? That would be like suddenly acting like a dead person's friend, just so you can soak up some sympathy and crash the funeral. Not only that, but it would be nice to recycle that name with a future baby. Tough times call for a bit of economizing.

Then there's the issue of whether to issue some kind of formal announcement of birth. Death. Dearth. Whatever. I was so looking forward to sending out little baby announcements when the time came. Why deprive myself of that fun chore?

"We should send out an announcement about the baby," I whisper to almost-sleeping Kevin one night. As usual, I'm lying awake in the darkness, obsessively adjusting the ice pack in my pajama bottoms and trying not to think too hard about anything meaningful. Sending out an announcement seems like a reachable and reasonable objective that— hopefully—wouldn't be upsetting or disturbing to others. Or would it? I have no idea, really. But again, how do you get by in a culture that doesn't have clear-cut rules about what to do, and what not to do? Once again: you bumble forward, making up your own rules as you go along. Maybe I'll start a new national trend. "What colors should we use?"

"Think of something creative," Kevin mumbles into his pillow. "That's your realm."

After another hour or so staring wide-awake into the darkness, I finally give up on sleeping. I pad into the office in my moose slippers and bathroom, and flip open my laptop, and search for an online card-design program. After carefully choosing a blue template design with little dragonflies flying in loops around the border, I type out a message in black, flowy font. With surprising effortlessness, the words from my brain down through my fingertips, straight onto the keyboard:

*Baby Boy LeMoine passed quickly through our lives in the early morning hours of Sunday, August 19th, 2007. He weighed 6 lbs, 1 oz., and had Irish brown hair and a gorgeous nose. In his eight months of life, our son knew only love and luxury:*

*A cozy womb with dim lighting,*
*A carte blanche to kick mom at random,*
*Unrestricted access to tasty amnio fluid,*
*Soothing voices of NPR announcers,*

*An occasional sweet taste of Pabst Blue Ribbon,*
*Lots of overpriced goodies from Whole Foods,*
*Knee and elbow massages by warm hands,*
*And pure love and excitement from many, many supporters.*
*Sweet little guy, you will live forever in the hearts of many.*

OKAY, I'LL ADMIT: I PRETTY MUCH MADE THAT WHOLE THING UP. Who am I to say if our baby lived in "love and luxury," or that amnio fluid is "tasty?" In fact, the entire process—choosing font styles and colors, ordering twenty-five of these printed note cards for sending to friends and family, entering my credit card information, clicking "submit"—feels rather like an empty corporate ritual, disconnected from the actual human baby that this announcement purportedly refers to.

Still, I find it oddly satisfying to see my finished piece of creative work, my words, my choice of color and font. Maybe this does pay our baby some vague form of respect, and maybe others will appreciate it. If nothing else, our little announcements will hopefully reassure everyone that Kevin and I are still alive and functioning human beings, capable of doing things like addressing and sending out note cards.

Hey World!
A boy was born
(I guess)

# HOME DEPOT THERAPY

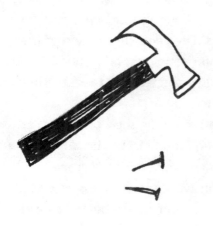

DO ALL MEN CHANNEL their grief into home repair projects? Because Kevin has developed a keen, sudden interest in finishing our half-started basement renovation project, and I'm wondering if this is normal. We had put it on hold because we didn't want non-baby-conducive paint fumes filling the house. Now that there isn't going to be a baby, Kevin points out, there couldn't be a better time to plow ahead and get the damn thing done, turning that basement into the party/recreation room of our dreams. Here's to child-free living! Normal or not, it sounds exciting, so I'm not going to argue.

We lie on the cool basement floor with our fingers interlocked, and Kevin lays out a plan of action. I just listen, watching his lips move and trying to fend off the black moroseness that's been lately closing in around my chest. He says he's going to pick up more Dry-Core tiles and finish the floor. He's also going to try to install track lighting by himself, since there's no reason he shouldn't be able to figure it out, and we'll have a contractor come in to install heaters. And—to top it off with style—we'll pick up a ping-pong table.

"That's great, but what am I gonna do this whole time?" I feel sulky, suddenly left out as Kevin explains all of this. "I mean, it pretty much sounds like you and the contractors have the whole thing covered."

"You get to make some paintings for the walls. Look how drab they are without any color. Where are your paints?"

"Dude, I don't know. We probably left them in Arkansas. Besides, even if they're around somewhere, I'm sure they're all dried up by now."

"I remember they got stuffed into a box before we left—let's find them. And if they're dried up we can buy new ones. I'll get you some canvas."

"I don't know what to paint."

"You'll think of something. You always do."

I guess I've never mentioned that I like to paint. It's a hobby that started decades ago, when my mom and I would draw murals on butcher paper and play "I tell you what to draw and you draw it." Back in Milwaukee, I painted city scenes on little pieces of paper and made greeting cards out of them, selling them at farmers' markets. But excitement over pregnancies began to overshadow excitement over painting, and all of my art supplies got put away for "later" when the artsy Monica returned, whenever "later" might be. Eighteen years later? "Later" must be right now, I suppose. I wish I felt more inspired by that fact. Kevin and I dig through the big Tupperware containers that we use for storage and find my now-dusty tubes of acrylic. I unscrew the cap of one of them and squeeze out a dollop of glistening orange paint, the heaviness of gloom lifting off me just a bit. This is something I *like* to do, I remember.

That same day, Kevin picks up four large stretched canvases on his way back from Home Depot. And so begins our all-day, home-improvement rampage: him snapping wooden pieces of flooring together, and me creating a series of brightly colored, thickly slathered paintings for the walls. Two gigantic flowers in orange and cobalt, with bright yellow centers and swirling green tendrils of stem and leaf. An enormous goldfish with flowy fins and black eyelashes, turquoise bubbles rising from her lips. We work in the basement in relative silence, each immersed in intense concentration, pausing occasionally to pee or rummage in the pantry for pistachios and Fritos. No time to cook dinner tonight. Ten hours later, after slanted evening sunlight has long passed across the dusty basement windows, we're stifling yawns and working from the light of bare bulbs hanging from the ceiling.

"Arright, I think I'm done for now," says Kevin. I look around for the first time, seeing our newly installed flooring more than half completed.

"Wow!" I say. "That looks awesome! Progress."

"You too. Three paintings—I'd say that's progress."

If that kid had worked out, I'd like to think he would have enjoyed having such progress-oriented parents. Even though this particular "progress" feels like a fake-plastic variety, I feel so pleased about it that I could just about cry.

# SEARCHING

THE PARTY FORMERLY KNOWN as the "Pre-Baby Dance Party" comes around, and everyone we know shows up for the affair—which we are now calling the "Pre-Halloween and New Basement Sub-Floor Celebration Dance Party." Same deal, different name.

Guests crowd into our dark and freshly sub-floored basement, where I've lit candles in strategic places for just the right atmosphere. The music thumps as I flit from person to person with a tray of Jello-shots, tossing my head back and laughing, pushing the booze like I always have. It seems easy and natural, being this person, or at least pretending to be—with my post-partum pudginess hidden beneath a baggy black t-shirt and face obscured in the darkness. This is hardly the time to have my physical appearance scrutinized from a close distance.

I chat with Jane and clink my glass of white wine against Nina and Carrie's sparkling cider, exchanging non-baby-related pleasantries while avoiding so much as an accidental glance at their now-huge bellies. Their due dates, what used to be "our" due dates, are coming up soon—a fact which really ought to make me feel disgusted with my life. But guess what: it doesn't! Through all of this mayhem, we're still friends. Hoorah! Aren't we?

When everyone has gone and my head is spinning from the cheap wine and vodka-infused Jello mingling in my stomach, Kevin and I plop down on the couch. He puts his arm around my shoulder and rests one hand on my thigh, squeezing gently.

"Hey," I say. "You're not allowed to touch my thighs until future notice."

"Why not?"

"Too fat. I'm like the Pillsbury doughboy. I feel fucking gross."

"You're ridiculous. So, I saw you over there talking to Nina and Carrie."

"Yeah." My voice falters at the tail end of that "yeah," and a fountain of sudden, seemingly random grief pushes up and out like lava from a volcano. I turn to Kevin and bury face into his armpit, crying in hard and quiet heaves.

He doesn't have to ask what's wrong. What's wrong is that talking to my prego-friends is like talking to an ex-boyfriend that you're still in love with: the more you converse with them, the lonelier you feel, because the huge, glaring gulf between you can't be ignored. What's wrong is that even having all these happy-making factors under one roof in a single evening—good friends, Jello-shots, pounding hip-hop, strung-up lights, booty shaking, a husband whose hand gravitates toward my thigh— doesn't fill the huge hole in my heart.

THERE ARE 3.2 MILLION STILLBIRTHS in the world each year, according to one of the many grief pamphlets floating around the house. I keep one of those pamphlets next to the toilet for bathroom reading, and when I see that number—3.2 million—I nearly fall off the warm seat.

*3.2 million??* That's a lot!

They must be out there somewhere, a whole sprawling tribe of stillbirth-mommas waiting for us to find one another so we can go out for coffee and have long, emotional conversations about our dead babies. Who needs Nina and Carrie! My people are around here somewhere, all 3.2 million of them. The question is how to find them.

I launch an Internet search for my stillbirth-mommy tribeswomen. What invariably pop up are memorial websites with headings like, "In Memory of Sweet Jonathan, Our Precious Perfect Angel Who Has Been Lifted Up Into the Arms of the Lord," coupled with sappy, depressing prose. Lots of pastel backgrounds and animated graphics, butterflies and bluebirds hopping from word to word, leaving looped trails that look like

118

bug-n-bird droppings behind them. Lots of teddy bears and kittens and ribbons. Some websites blast Celine Dion-esque music, which causes me to breathe in sharply and frantically search for the "mute" button. Of course, I can never seem to find it before Kevin calls out from three rooms away: "What the hell was *that*?"

Busted.

The problem is, I don't even *like* sappy things, sentimental things, religious things, pink and purple things, girly things, Celine Dion-esque things. And what? Losing a baby means I suddenly have to be all into teddy bears and Jesus? After several days of fruitless searching for connection, I wind up feeling worse, not better. I'm a wandering, tribeless nomad, outcast from just about every group on the planet: my baby-having friends. Other stillbirth mommies. Single friends who can't possibly imagine what it's like to carry a child to term.

Dude, I am so screwed.

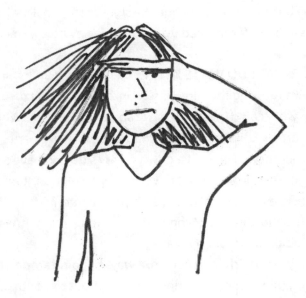

# Becoming a Boy

"DO YOU THINK WE SHOULD start calling him Zachary?" We're driving home from the sporting-goods store, where we spent the last hour perusing ping-pong tables. "All the grief pamphlets say it's a good idea, so we might want to try it. I mean, not in front of other people—that would be weird. Just between us."

"Sure, if you want," says Kevin.

"Okay. Here, I'll try it: Zachary. Zachary LeMoine."

Just a name, nothing else. I whisper it again. *Zachary, Zachary, Zachary.* It doesn't make me feel noticeably better about anything—further confirming my suspicion that grief pamphlets are full of shit. Sniffling, I stare glumly out the window, hating the sight of strip malls whizzing past, the grayness, the traffic stacked up on the freeway below the railing.

HERE'S WHAT I DO WHILE KEVIN'S OFF doing manly things around the house, like mowing the yard, or scrutinizing our credit card bill online, wondering who could possibly have spent $106.72 at Whole Foods, because it sure as hell wasn't *him*. I grab a roll of toilet paper and sneak off into the bedroom, where I lie down on my side and have a good hard cry. Although I revel in those first few minutes in solitude, it isn't very long before I send Kevin a telepathic message to come find me. What's the point of just lying there sobbing with no one to enjoy it with? It's like publishing a blog that nobody reads.

Normally, I'm a fairly loud person, always banging around the kitchen and dropping things and chattering to Kevin about this or that. You won't find me off in a hidden corner with my nose in a book. So when the house is abruptly quiet, Kevin really does notice it. He stops whatever he's doing and makes his way into the bedroom (he somehow just knows I'm there), slides up onto the bed beside me, and drapes his arm across my torso.

Through a blurry film of tears, I look up at his face, which to me is absolutely perfect. Symmetrical features. Sandpaper scruff. Dark eyebrows. And his face inevitably morphs into what Zachary's face would look like, grown up. Once I get that hurtful image in my head, I can't erase it, so I press my face against Kevin's chest instead and close my eyes. I then attempt to breathe in his scent through the long-sleeve t-shirt he always wears, for he's got that summer boy smell I love—sweaty and salty and outdoorsy and clean. But by that time, of course, both of my nostrils are totally clogged—so I end up sucking down my own snot through my back nasal passage instead.

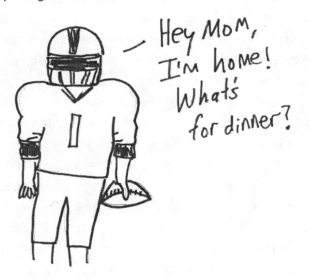

Hey MOM, I'm home! What's for dinner?

I then try to imagine that scent, which I can always do with great accuracy, and wonder why men's cologne companies can never seem to hit the mark. It's precisely what Zachary would have smelled like as a buff young high school student, bursting through the front door after football practice with sweaty armpits and grass-stained knees, alive and flushed and filled with vitality. He would have opened the fridge and grabbed the entire carton of two-percent milk and started chugging it, in that impulsive teenage boy kind of way. And then, he would have joined Kevin and me at the dinner table, where we would have eaten something simple and weeknighty. Not Hamburger Helper, since the eighties are totally over, but maybe stir-fried tofu and curried vegetables with rice. Zach would most certainly grow up to be a vegetable lover, unafraid of spicy or exotic foods, having spent several years of his youth in Bangladesh or Guatemala, wherever Kevin and I had dragged him to do international teaching or volunteering stints. He might even be one of several kids in the family, but I can't think about that now.

I turn away from Kevin and stare at the ceiling, tears pouring out in rivulets, again flowing straight into my ears. By this point, my wad of toilet paper is totally saturated with snot and spit and disintegrating in the palm of my hand, but I hardly notice. Kevin is upset too, I can just feel it in the warmth of his body, the way he's breathing shakily, the force with which he's clamping down on me, wishing he was in control.

And then Kevin and I have a simple conversation: me proclaiming that I want my son, unable to mask the despair and hurt that I feel. Kevin assuring me that he knows, he misses our son too. Me repeating with increased agitation that I want my son. Kevin saying nothing at all, just taking a deep breath and pressing against me. It's frustrating to talk in circles like this, pining after something that no longer exists, something that Kevin can't produce for me with a few magic words. Kind of like trying to hug the air, hoping my arms will land on my baby boy, alive and wiggling around and looking up at me, and always coming up empty.

Once we've gone back and forth about this to my satisfaction, once I feel certain that I have sufficiently and accurately conveyed my main point, once my snot and tear reserves are depleted and I've had it with all this fruitless blubbering, I ask Kevin to tell me a funny Chuck Farting Story. I'm talking, of course, about his old college roommate Chuck, who had undiagnosed but seriously nasty gas problems. One of my favorite tales is when Chuck and Kevin and some other people went to Las Vegas, and Chuck ate so many beans at a Tex-Mex buffet that he turned the entire hotel room into a stench cube that night, and Kevin had to go sleep out in the hall. I know Kevin thinks it's silly to force such contrived, inorganic discourse—the good stories should come up naturally, he always tells me—but nowadays, thankfully, he goes along with it.

We end with good belly laugh, and Kevin's relieved that I'm not going to slit my wrists, and I'm relieved that he's not going to slit his wrists, not that I was ever concerned about that, and he's relieved that I'm relieved. And then we just get on with our day like nothing out of the ordinary happened.

## SPRUCING UP

KEVIN AND I ARE SITTING at the small wooden table on the deck, slurping down the last drops of coffee out of great big mugs. I'm in an oddly upbeat mood. Could be the coffee, or the blissfully cool morning weather.

"How're you feeling this morning?" says Kevin. "You look good."

"Fine, actually. Much, much better than yesterday." I lean back in my chair, closing my eyes and raising my arms toward the sky to stretch. "I can't believe I'm starting work in, like, a week-and-a-half!"

"Yup," Kevin says, nodding. "I'm gonna go weed-whack the yard." He pushes back from the table and stands up.

"But wait! We're, like, having a conversation!"

"I thought we were done. Besides, the lawn looks like crap."

He's right. I know full well that our rapidly browning, overgrown yard needs some serious tender loving care, and I ought to go help him. But I tell Kevin that my first morning calling is to take inventory of my work-appropriate wardrobe. Dead baby or no dead baby, I do have a professional image to uphold, after all, starting with my clothes!

I trot down the basement steps and pick up the gigantic plastic storage container in which all of my pre-pregnancy work clothes are kept. It's covered in a film of dust and red droplets of spilled paint from when Kevin went on his mad post-stillbirth basement-ceiling-painting bonanza. I lug it upstairs and dump out its contents, which fall onto the bed like a solid brick of compacted clothing, retaining the shape of the container itself. It quickly becomes apparent that my pre-pregnancy outfits are several sizes too small—I can tell without going through the agony of trying to stuff myself into them. So I rummage through my dresser drawers for some larger sizes, only to find that everything I own is either frumpy or ill-fitting or both. I wasn't planning to actually look good in all those drab maternity clothes from garage sales.

For the first time in weeks, I look at myself in the mirror. I mean, really give myself a good up-and-down stare in full lighting. My light blue tank top, which I've been sleeping in without washing since I returned home from the hospital, is stained in various places with residual booby milk, snot, tears, spit, and coffee. My hair, which I haven't brushed in weeks, is a long, tangled mop. Just for kicks, I grab Kevin's blue plastic hairbrush, press it against the top of my head and attempt to pull it downward, but it's immediately stopped by a monster-sized knot. So much for that idea. I then notice that my forehead is breaking out, and the line etched in my skin between my nose and the left corner of my mouth seems more pronounced, and my teeth look yellow.

You know what? It's officially time to spruce up my appearance and quit being such a slob, especially since I'm about to begin teaching three sections of college writing. How on earth are my students, or anyone else for that matter, going to respect me when I look like I've been living in a cave for the past year? I shove all of my old clothing—anything that doesn't instantly inspire me—into a corner of the room and remind myself to drive it to the Goodwill later. Then, after peeling off my stained tank top and tossing it into the laundry hamper, I slip on a clean pair of maternity jeans and one of Kevin's t-shirts—a nice baggy one that hides the paunch. Grabbing my purse and wallet, I yell out the window that I'm off to run a few errands. Kevin tells me not to spend too much, and I tell him of course I won't. I'm the frugal Peace Corps type, remember?

My first stop is Great Clips, the one in the strip mall by our house. I tell the gum-chewing girl at the front desk that I'd like a haircut, something short and cute. So she hacks off about six inches of brown knots, all the way up to the nape of my neck, and gives my hair some feathery layers. I walk out feeling like I'm off to a good start.

Then, I go into Target and head straight for the toiletries section, which is brimming with lotions, astringent liquids and sprays designed to make women feel more beautiful. After carefully perusing the shelves, I settle on Stridex medicated pads for zits, Ponds Cold Cream for facial wrinkles, Colgate Whitening Toothpaste, a shiny new tube of Great Lash mascara in jet black, and a bottle of chewable Vitamin C tablets—which I figure must be good for something.

Next stop is JC Penny for dressy tops and skirts. To my dismay, I find that I have to do some serious sucking-in-the-stomach in order to fit into a size six like I used to be able to. So I settle on a few things in different sizes—one for the "now" me, and one for the "after I start jogging again" me—and a pair of fake-pearl earrings for a touch of glamour.

On the way out, I pop into the Gap, only to do a quick search through the sales rack, of course, but end up leaving with two absolutely must-have, albeit non-sale, items: a brown sweater-wrap that ties around the waist, and a satin-lined corduroy jacket. So scholarly and stylish looking, perfect for a college writing teacher! Kevin and God will surely forgive me for dropping two hundred bucks on mass-produced clothing from Chinese sweatshops, just this once.

I arrive home satisfied with my purchases and new look, and waste no time in trying everything on again and parading through the living room to show it off for Kevin. I ask him several times if he likes my new haircut, and he consistently says "yes." He doesn't even ask me how much it all cost. Better for him not to know.

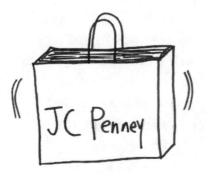

# Dipping a Toe in the Real World

SUMMER VACATION OFFICIALLY reaches its end, and it's time for both of us to return to work. No more sitting lazily around the house, working in the peaceful basement, feeling alternately fine and not fine, gorging ourselves on the endless stream of casseroles that continue to land on our front porch. On my first morning back to work, I feel a mixture of excitement and anxiety. This is familiar territory, I remind myself as I vigorously rub Burt's Bees lotion into the crow's feet around my eyes. Unlike making babies, teaching is something I do—and have done—with relative success. No need to worry.

After changing outfits five different times, not even liking the way my body fits into my recent mall-purchases, I finally settle on khaki pants (not fully buttoned up), a flowery blouse, and my good old, paunch-swallowing Hanes undies. My newly short hair is pinned back with clips to show that I take my professional appearance seriously, with just enough loose strands falling into my face to keep me from looking overly prim. I wear heels for added height—not dressy mile-high heels that might scare my students into permanent writer's block, but slightly dressy loafer type shoes from the Walking Store. The kind of shoes that shout, "I'm super easy-going! Now write me your very best essay!"

I arrive at my office building and offer light, airy good-mornings to the secretary and other instructors passing by, bracing myself to be pulled aside by someone and told some hushed words of condolence. Nobody does, which I suppose is a good thing for the sake of keeping composure. With a stack of course syllabi balanced on one arm like someone who has done it a million times before, I stride into my first period class, smile broadly, and greet my young students.

Despite my earnest efforts to look and act calm, to say uproariously funny things, I am greeted with an unending sea of silent teenage-and-twenty-something stares. And as the week progresses, I frantically rifle through my repertoire of exciting things to do in class—debates, teamwork, games, computer tricks, discussions on the most wacky pop culture topics I can think of—and yet I can't seem to draw their attention away from the clock above the door or the cell phones hidden in their laps. When they do look at me, although I want in my heart of hearts for it to be with inspiration and awe, I sense that it's more with apathy, irritation, sleepiness. Or worse, if this is even possible, hateful recognition of my reproductive failures and bodily flab.

This makes me wonder if I've forgotten how to teach, if I've chosen the wrong career altogether. Which is more than a little disturbing to ponder.

If I don't have this, then what the hell do I have?

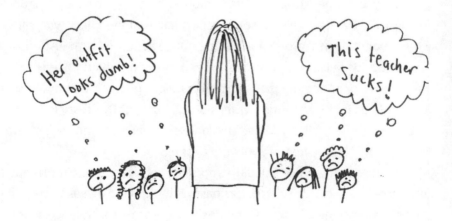

# CRACK IN THE SNOW GLOBE

BACK ON THAT FATEFUL DAY in the hospital, one of the first people I called was Jane. I needed some girlfriend-perspective.

"Jane, we're gonna lose the baby."

"WHAT?"

I explained the details as she inhaled sharply with disbelief, uttering a string of sorrowful profanity that mirrored my own thoughts. Things like *hell* and *fuck* and *isn't there anything they can do* and *how could this happen* and *I can't believe it* and *are you sure* and *holy shit*. It soothed me to hear someone so upset on my behalf. I told her to call the others.

Jane didn't have to ask who I meant by "the others." She would immediately phone both Nina and Carrie, I knew, and relay the news in a grave voice. More than any other friends, the three of them would mourn for me, for Kevin, for the baby. They would understand right away the profound implications this event was to have on our friendships, our much-fantasized-about journeys into new parenthood together. I would be excluded from this journey now, spiraling off on a weird, unexplored path of my own.

I had a vague sense of this from the beginning, from how I felt when they all showed up with flowers and food, faces puffy from their own grieving. It was this odd mixture of comfort combined with searing loneliness, as though I was now seeing them from the other side of some invisible glass wall that couldn't be traversed, no matter how hard we all banged our bruised fists against it. And then, just before the dance party, I sensed it again as I was sitting at the kitchen table in my pajamas, digging away at a bowl of Grape Nuts with milk. With my battle-against-the-boobs officially over, I had now become focused instead on small, meaningless tasks. Tasks like pushing my Grape Nuts to one side of the bowl in the shape of a crescent, patting it down to make it more symmetrical, and then carving out a bite from the crescent's tip with my spoon. It was right then, in the midst of sculpting my Grape Nuts, that I realized with great horror and crystal clarity: Nina and Carrie, although shocked and saddened by our news, would—in all likelihood—go on to have their babies, and continue to have a special, new-mommy friendship together. Without *me*, that is. Me, of all people! The one who introduced them! And what was to stop Jane from having another baby herself? Nothing! There was simply no end to the possible ways in which I could be left behind. This was unacceptable.

I pushed back from the table, milk sloshing up to the edge my bowl, and ran outside to the back gate as tiny pebbles stuck to the bottoms of my bare feet. Kevin poked his head out from the entrance to our sagging clapboard garage, where he had been tinkering with his bicycle all morning. There was a black smudge of chain grease on his cheek. I must have had a panicked look on my face.

"You alright?" he said.

"Carrie and Nina are supposed to have their babies…like…soon! How are we going to still be friends with them?" My eyes filled up with tears as I stood there, pajama bottoms billowing outward in the breeze. Kevin disappeared into the garage again and I heard him setting his tools down on the workbench. Then he came back out, wiping his palms on the fronts of his shorts, and put his arms around me.

"It's gonna be tricky, but I think we can still be friends. We'll just have to make that first move, and let them know that we still wanna hang out. You're good at that."

There he went again, reminding me of how I was. How I *used* to be, anyway—as if any elements of my former self still applied in this strange new reality. Still, I'd have to take Kevin's word for it, and trust myself to keep these friendships together. I had no choice, really, because the thought of being excluded, of my little snow-globe world of prego-friends and happiness disappearing, was more than I could bear. Staring back down at my soggy Grape Nuts, I vowed through gritted teeth to keep my pre-dead-baby world, the world I'd worked so hard to build, from draining away.

THE BREATHLESS CALL COMES from Bruce first. I am standing at the porcelain kitchen sink with a soapy dish in my hand when the phone rings. *Baby Carly has arrived! Carrie and baby are doing just fine!* The news, although not unexpected, feels like a hammer against my carefully constructed snow-globe world. Nina and David's nine-pound baby Damon follows and it's an unfamiliar voice on the other end of the phone this time—some friend of Nina's I've never met. Not that Nina would ever ask me, of all people, to call everyone in the world to announce her son's birth. Still, it bothers me that I'm not "that friend," the one at the top of the phone tree. I'd like to think I would have been that friend, could have been. In both cases, Kevin and I are among the first to pay a hospital visit. To not visit them, just because of my own less-than-happy ending, would make me feel even more alienated. Wouldn't it?

The visits themselves, although weeks apart, feel nearly identical. Both begin with me casting Kevin all sorts of meaningful looks, searching for some acknowledgement of how hard this is, some recognition of what a big person I must look like for doing it, yet avoiding actually saying those words: *this is hard*. Both involve us circling blocks to look for parking, a freight train of nervous adrenaline running through my head. Both involve stepping into an elevator and pressing a lit-up number, exiting into a dimly lit hallway with anti-septic smelling air, and knocking gently on a numbered door. Both involve getting greeted by Bruce and David respectively, and each have that frazzled, jacked-up, heavy-eyed appearance of college students who just pulled all-nighters. There are lots of soft-voiced hellos and hugs, passing the quiet and swaddled newborn from person to person, a warm and heavy little body against my chest. Both times, I think about Zachary and how he felt in my arms. Unnervingly similar to this, yet ghoulishly and depressingly different. And both times, congratulatory words come out of my mouth, clipped and faster than usual.

Everything feels wrong and fake, my words and body language forced, my happiness all pretend. This isn't how real friends are supposed to act and feel toward one another. It's my first indication that a very real fracture is creeping across my happy snow-globe-world; that these carefully cultivated and much-worshiped relationships are changing beyond my control.

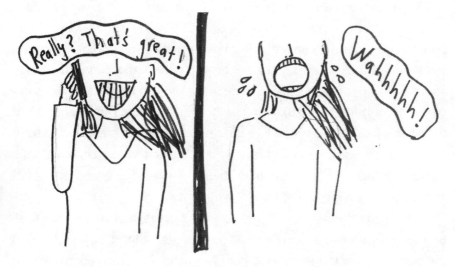

Or maybe I've just been harboring a secret and horrible hope, way deep down in the black corner of my heart where my most shameful thoughts click around like cockroaches, that one of *their* babies might be stillborn too, so that I wouldn't feel so freakish and alone. But I never admit this notion to anyone, because of course it isn't something I would *really* hope for. It might just make me feel temporarily better in a twisted way, like binging whiskey shots and puking the next day, feeling like total crap in the end.

# CRATE-N-BARREL BABY

I JUST CAN'T DO IT. A baby-less life of exclusion from the Baby Ladies—as I've begun to call Nina, Carrie and Jane—is decidedly not okay. Whoever sent me this unwanted life, come and get it back, or it's going straight into the dumpster. The question is no longer about how to adapt to this new reality, but how to ditch it and catch up with the Baby Ladies on their parenthood journeys. I could get pregnant again ASAP, but that process hasn't shown itself to be a guaranteed solution. Screw that: I'm looking for the money shot.

There is one money shot that has been brewing in my mind for several days now. It's a plan that, if executed properly, will result in a real, wiggling, live baby to call my own. Best of all, it will only require three things:

• About $30,000 (we can surely scrape together that amount in savings, supplemented by a no-interest "loan" from our parents);

• A plethora of paperwork and lengthy interviews (these things certainly didn't stop me from getting into the Peace Corps, attending graduate school, or being offered my current job—so why should they stop me now!); and

• Acceptance of a substitute child in place of my own. This step will likely be the most challenging—but where there's a will, there's a way. And there is no shortage of will around here.

It's called…drum roll please….adoption, which is similar to the (P)enis + (V)agina = (B)aby method of baby-making that has worked so well for others, except that (P)enis + (V)agina is replaced with (P)en + (V)at of

*Money*. The beauty of it all is that both equations have the same end result: *(B)aby*. Easy!

Time wise, adoption is a near-perfect solution. If we begin the adoption process now, it will probably be a year at least before we get a kid, who I imagine will be close to a year old at that time—putting me and my baby right up there with the Baby Ladies and theirs. Sure, I'll miss the first year or so of the new-parenthood action, but that's okay. I can wait.

Kevin, of course, is a major part of the equation as well. In fact, the true equation should read: *(P)en + (V)at of Money + (S)pousal Agreement = (B)aby*. I bring it up one day as we're on the futon in my favorite position: me lying down with my bare feet on his lap.

"What about adoption?"

He looks up from his book. "I think we should wait. It's only been… what…a few months?"

"But, adoption is perfect, because you just pay the money, sign the papers, and boom—you get your baby at the end. They probably refund your money if it doesn't work out."

"I doubt it's that simple."

"No, it is! I've already researched it!" Not really true, but it sounds convincing. "Kev, look. I want a baby, and the sooner we have one, the sooner we catch up with the Baby Ladies, and the sooner our kid will be grown up and off to college. And then we can join the Peace Corps again as retirees! My parents will help us with the adoption fees, you know they will."

"I guess we could at least look into it down the line sometime," he finally says, presumably to put an end to this conversation.

"Down the line" for me means that very same afternoon, so I brew a pot of coffee and dive straight into the Internet, frantically looking for adoption agencies. My caffeine-fueled search continues every day for the next week while Kevin is away at work. Never mind that stacks of students' essays have yet to be graded, my mother has left six fretful voicemail messages that haven't been returned, my armpits are looking like a wooly mammoth's, the living room is a mess, we're almost out of milk, and my eyelids are heavy from permanent exhaustion. No time to nap or pay attention to such trivial matters of human life; I'm a mother in search of my motherhood!

I stumble across people's personal websites, called things like: "Life with Lily, Our Adopted Chinese Baby," "Journey to Guatemala for Our Son, Griffin." Like a voyeur, I scroll through their pictures and try to imagine myself in their shoes, their babies as mine. I post bold, enthusiastic announcements on blogs and forums: *"I'm planning to adopt too, and I'm so excited! Anyone with tips or insight, please let me know!"*

Thick, glossy packets from places like "All God's Children" and "Americans Adopting Orphans" are sent to us in droves, stacking up on the coffee table like Crate and Barrel catalogs. Sleekly organized and brimming with photos and charts, they all begin with a blurb on whether adoption is "right for you," and allot several pages to each country. China. India. Kazakhstan. Ethiopia. Russia.

Flipping through these booklets is a bit like shopping for a new car or a custom-built home plan: for granite countertops and bamboo floors, go with Model C. Some include lists of "no wait list" children, available right away or for a lower fee because of being older or having a disability. A heart defect here, a missing limb there. A zit-faced teenager from Romania. These kids are advertised boldly in red font, like Thanksgiving Day sale items in the Nordstrom catalog: "Adoption fees waived! No wait time!"

EVERYTHING LOOKS SO EASY: choose your features, hand over the cash, and a baby will be shipped to your doorstep via FedEx, complete with a day's supply of diapers and a half-off coupon for your next baby. I wonder if, perhaps, I could credit some of my unused frequent flyer miles toward the purchase of a new son. Adoption seems so convenient, in fact, that I can't help but wonder why anyone bothers to go about baby-having in the sloppy, vagina-stretching, back-aching, shitting-yourself, old fashioned way.

Since this is Kevin's life too, I drag him to an adoption fair in the rain. It's a long, dreary drive into the bowels of suburbia. The room is lined with booths, each with a suit-clad representative of an adoption agency or law firm, ready to chat and give out butterscotch candies. This is serious business, so I linger at each table, collecting armloads of information, eavesdropping on others' conversations, and discussing adoption logistics with lawyers and ...what would you call them...baby salespeople?

Kevin, on the other hand, spins through in about sixty seconds, conveniently settling into a comfy chair in the lobby, next to the coffee-and-cookie table. Like one of those dads slumped in a leather chair at the mall while his wife does the shopping, he waits patiently—and I eventually stagger toward them with a foot-tall stack of brochures and packets in my arms. I feel a twinge of mild irritation with him for not taking this crucial event more seriously. On the other hand, I know it's not his fault for not understanding that this fair—as a key stepping stone toward getting our baby—should be approached with seriousness. He is a man, after all, and men don't get things like this.

I begin filling out application forms, but—after a week or so—get distracted with other things and set the paperwork aside. Now that I think about it, none of those babies in the catalogs really sounds appealing to me. Knowing my luck, whatever kid we adopted would probably act like a total shit head, unlike our quiet little perfect boy, Zachary. What I really want, I finally come to realize, is *my* baby, the one who isn't here—a mysterious fact which still perplexes me to no end. There is no substitute model, no quick fix, no swapping tofu for chicken and not noticing it, no buying a K-mart brand handbag and slapping a Gucci label on it. So the Crate and Barrel baby catalogs begin to gather dust, and eventually get stacked up and tossed into the bedroom closet. *Oh, well, it was a nice thought.*

# HALF MOM, HALF NOT

ON THE SURFACE, THINGS seem back to business as usual. The familiar city skyline: unchanging and visible from the hill at the top of our street, etched against Seattle's perpetual cloud cover. Traffic: characteristically everywhere, slow-moving lines of cars snaking up to intersections and crawling along the interstate. Slimy green moss: drooping from the roof of our clapboard garage. Kevin: shaving, showering, coming home at night, programming the coffee maker before bed, writing out checks to pay bills. Friends and family members: calling with decreased frequency, working, living their lives. Nina and Carrie: raising their new babies, I imagine. We haven't talked much lately. Me: driving along the freeway; cramming my yogurt into the office fridge and hoping it doesn't get eaten by the office-fridge gremlins; sitting in faculty meetings, teaching my unnervingly quiet writing classes, and wondering what I'm doing wrong.

Somehow, though, all of this seems like a mere template of a life, nothing more. I feel stuck in the past, stagnant, unable to pinpoint exactly what's broken or unresolved. Oh, I could keep poring over the grief literature, maybe drop in on the local support group in search of answers, but it kind of feels like I've been there, done that. Already gleaned whatever rare and insightful suggestions those Ph.D-holding authors and facilitators have to offer. What I need right now is something concrete to launch us to the next segment in life, whatever that might be. This segment blows.

Another pregnancy, perhaps. Maybe that's the ticket. I begin pressing my body against Kevin's in the middle of the night in an effort to instigate sex. My heart isn't in it, though, because I feel just flabby and gross.

IT'S NEARLY TEN O'CLOCK AT NIGHT, and Kevin isn't home from work yet, as usual. I'm standing at the kitchen sink in my flannel pajamas, hair up in a sloppy ponytail, scrubbing dishes and chatting with my brother Paul on the cordless phone. I'm glad he called, for I've been in a dark mood all evening, thinking about babies. My head is cocked to one side in order to keep the phone balanced on my shoulder, and several times it almost falls into the sudsy water.

"So, I've been meaning to ask you, are you guys gonna try again for a baby anytime soon?" says Paul.

Funny he should ask. Just yesterday morning before the sun came up, I pressed my frontside against Kevin's in hopes of arousing him for that very purpose—but he just groaned in that half-asleep way and burrowed deeper into his pillow. Which, naturally, confirmed my nervous suspicion that I'm turning into a sexually unattractive lard-ass.

"I want to, yeah." The answer tumbles from my mouth without hesitation. "Soon as we can."

"Hmmm," says Paul. "Have you given any thought to just...taking a break from having babies? It seems like you've been really focused on getting pregnant the past few years. What about cooling it for a while?"

"Cooling it?"

"Like, giving yourselves the next year or two to just...do the things you want to do together without worrying about having a baby. You know, traveling overseas and backpacking and stuff. You live in such an awesome city, so why not get out and enjoy it? Or you could start your painting back up again. Just to reconnect with who you really are."

*Reconnect with who I really am?*

"Mmmm, I see what you're saying," I say. "I'll think about it." *Not.*

Hanging up the phone, I dry my hands and head into the bathroom to brush my teeth. Kevin comes in through the back door and finds me there, kissing me lightly on the neck.

"Hi."

"Hi. How was prison today?"

"Oh, the usual. It's good to be out."

"I talked to Paul just a few minutes ago. He's fine. He said something about maybe taking a break for a while before we try for another baby. What do you think about that?"

"I think he's totally right."

*"Really?"* Opening my mouth wide, I strain to jam floss between my back molars. "What are we supposed to do with our lives for the next few years if we're not...like...trying for a baby?" My words sound garbled. Note to self: flossing and talking simultaneously doesn't work so well.

"Let's talk about it tomorrow, Mon. I gotta get some sleep."

That night, I'm kept awake by mind-chatter. This seems to be happening a lot lately. I drink an extra coffee in the afternoon; hardly sleep a wink at night; then need even more caffeine the following day just to get by without falling asleep in front of students. Paul's words replay themselves in my mind as I stare at the black ceiling.

*Reconnect with who you are.*

*Who I am,* or who I've been for the past two years anyway, is a pregnant woman (or trying-to-get pregnant woman)—eating, breathing, and living for two. According to everything I've read and heard, a dead-baby momma is still a momma. And real mommas don't do things like traveling and painting. Okay, so I don't have a baby to call my own—but I see no reason to start running around doing childfree things. You don't drop out of medical school and become a plumber, just because you fail a quiz or two (or in this case, the final exam).

Still, I keep going back to the problem of not having an actual kid in tow. I'm not about to become the person who carries around a framed picture of Zachary and talks to it, showing up for mommy groups with it wrapped in a blanket and introducing it as my son, while the other women look at me with sad sympathy. *Poor, delusional Monica. She thinks she's a Real Mom.*

I slide my hand underneath my flannel pajama top and feel my belly, which still boasts a distinct paunch of flab that I halfheartedly assure myself is a postpartum side effect. No movement underneath that paunch, no distinct presence of baby limbs all squished up inside of me anymore. It's quite possible that the grief literature has been lying to me all along, telling me I'm a mother just to make me feel better. It's condescending, sort of like agreeing with everything an Alzheimer's patient says no matter how off-the-wall it is. "Yes, Monica, that picture of a baby is your child. Don't worry about him not talking or moving at all; he's kind of an introvert."

Logically, I know there is no damned kid, and yet I can't seem to let it go of that life, that notion of myself. It's all I've had these past few years. A couple of warm tears prick at my eyes and seep out. I briefly consider blowing my nose as hard as I can on a piece of toilet paper just to jolt Kevin from sleep, "accidentally" waking him up for input. But I decide not to dip into what I feel are my limited quota of times that I can roust him from slumber to chat about depressing, pointless topics in the middle of the night.

A mother or not a mother: I'll just keep this little conundrum private, and hope it works itself out.

## ASHES ON MY HANDS

IT'S BEEN ABOUT TWO MONTHS since Dr. Williams looked at me gravely with furrowed brows. There's still a hugely important detail to take care of, and it's not something we're doing because a big corporation or anyone else is compelling us. Nobody is telling us anything useful on this self-guided stillbirth tour, remember? So Kevin and I continue to act on instinct, which has led us in a great big circle. Off to the distracting battle against the boobs, the frenzied basement projects, the midnight card-designing sprees, the adoption catalogs, and now—finally—back to the core fact in front that's been sitting in front of us all along: *we loved the baby, and now he's gone.*

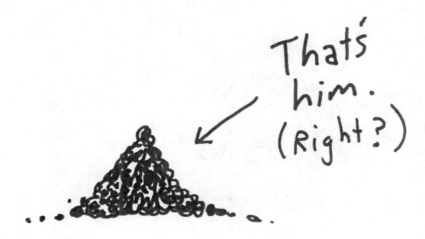

It's 7:30 a.m. on a dark Sunday morning. Steel-colored clouds hang low over the city as sheets of rain hit the windows and rooftops. Theoretically,

I've accomplished a lot since 6 a.m. when I woke up and bolted upright in bed, staring wide-eyed into the darkness:

- Took a long, steaming-hot shower. Shaved my legs and armpits and bikini line, tapping the razor's edge on the ceramic tiled wall to be wiped away later by Kevin (he loves it).
- Slammed a mug of coffee.
- In a fury of caffeine-induced energy, Windexed the counter tops and brass ledge above the fireplace. Peered at the satisfying strip of black dust left on the moist paper towel, feeling momentarily tidy and productive.
- Threw on a sweatshirt over my other sweatshirt, pulled rubber rain boots onto my feet, and drove through the empty, blue-lit streets to the bakery as rain slid down the windshield.
- Picked up several dozen assorted bagels and plastic tubs of cream cheese, zipped home while blasting "Video Killed the Radio Star," and drummed my cold fingers to the beat.
- Arrived home and arranged bagels in pyramid shapes on large ceramic plates.

And all of this I accomplished being relatively quiet—which is a remarkable feat for me—so as not to wake up Mom and my brother Paul, who are visiting for a few days.

Now, having come down from that early morning energy rush, I'm sitting sullenly on the edge of the bed in my bra and Hanes underwear, my bare feet dangling over the floor, head resting in my hands. Kevin is rummaging around in the closet, pulling out dresses on hangers.

"How 'bout this?" he says, handing me the ankle-length, blue cotton sundress from Talbot's, the one I used to wear on hot summer days in Uzbekistan. "I like you in this one."

I know he likes it. That's why I've kept it all these years, even though the color has faded and the strings in the back are frayed. I still recall the way my stomach did a joyful forward flip when he first told me, "I like you in that dress," lowering his mouth over mine. Now, though, I shake my head ruefully.

"It doesn't fit anymore. Makes me look fat, like whatever you'd call a muffin-top for your upper arms. Besides, it's too cold for that dress."

Nothing fits. Nothing works. Nothing I own is appropriate for a memorial in the rain, for meandering out onto the chilly, seaweed-and-shell-covered beach and throwing my infant son's ashes into the headlong wind, ducking as they inevitably blow back toward my face. Nothing is the right color, the right style. Nothing will comfortably zip or snap, make my postpartum body fat disappear.

God, I hate my body. Hate it, hate it, hate it. When I stand in the shower and look down, I only see pasty white belly flab, a washed out dead baby factory. Insert sperm, wait a while, and out shoots a lifeless entity on a conveyor belt. Not exactly a thong-worthy object d'art, a body worth screwing or even caressing. And I'm not even going to go into the upper arm fat, which serves absolutely no discernable, biological purpose during pregnancy, and therefore must have come from all the full-fat milk and cheeseburgers I've been eating. Purely my food-loving fault.

"Arright," says Kevin. "Wear this and a sweater over it." A command, not a suggestion. Fine with me. It's what I need sometimes—being bossed around, like that military commando nurse who somehow made me deliver my dead son. Kevin hands me a long, brown summer dress with a blue floral print, flowy and mermaid-like with lacy shoulder straps. This one I wore in Mexico, sipping cocktails on the moonlit beach and rubbing my foot along Kevin's hairy calf. Seems kind of twisted to be wearing this now, but whatever.

I sigh and squeeze into it, almost busting the zipper in the back; pull on a mercifully baggy cardigan sweater; haphazardly drag a wand of black mascara across my lashes; and slip my feet into my ratty old summer sandals. I don't care if my feet are going to freeze or I look like a bag lady. Kevin is wearing something nice; I can't focus on exactly what that nice thing is. A suit, maybe, or khaki pants and a collared shirt. Something respectful of the moment.

Mom and Paul are awake now and padding around the house. I go out and say my good mornings. We exchange our typical familial pleasantries, pouring coffee refills and rehashing how many guests will be at the post-memorial brunch in our living room. Mom busily cuts oranges and apples into cubes for a fruit salad, and my brother retreats to the futon, scrawling something hastily on a notepad. His opening speech, I presume. The morning news is on the kitchen radio, but nobody seems to be listening.

After everyone has brushed and preened and finished our last drops of coffee, we grab raincoats and wallets, and I scoop up Zachary's two framed photographs. They seem like an appropriate thing to bring. We all dash outside and crowd into the tan Buick. On the way, I impulsively stop to pluck a tiny purple flower from one of the weed-like bushes in the yard, and stick it behind my ear. It makes me feminine and motherly. Don't little boys get a kick out of flowers in their mothers' hair? Wouldn't Zachary enjoy it if he were here? I would think so.

We drive west toward the Puget Sound, Kevin in the drivers' seat, everybody commenting on the dismal weather, not talking directly about the grim event that is the centerpiece of the morning. I feel hollow inside as pine trees whiz past in the damp morning grayness.

Ten minutes later, we arrive at Carkeek Park, a place etched in my childhood memory. My parents and Paul and I used to come here often, to this narrow swath of dark and sandy beach, littered with shells and dead crab carcasses, long ropes of slimy seaweed and jagged hunks of driftwood, tidal pools teeming with spiny and rubbery-looking creatures. Reaching the water's edge required crossing over the train tracks on a high, metal bridge, and Paul and I used to lean over it and spit on the trains roaring by. The metal bridge is still there, just as it was when I was eight years old, and so are the train tracks.

Not every friend and family member is here, and Dad stayed in St. Louis because he wasn't feeling well. This isn't a real funeral that people are actually expected to *attend*, I assured everyone; more just a casual, come-if-you-can sort of affair. Funerals are for bona fide humans who once had publicly recognizable lives. *This*, on the other hand, is just a memorial-esque ritual, a way to make the loss of Zachary more official, perhaps even bring some closure. It was mostly my idea to do this (not even really my idea, but something one of the grief pamphlets told me I should do), and Kevin agreed it would be worthwhile.

A small crowd of people has gathered there to wait for us, clamoring around under umbrellas. I see Nina and David, without the baby, and Jane and Jayson. Some of my parents' friends are there, older people in their fifties and sixties, looking calmer than the younger folks, having been around the block. *Yup, this shit happens*, I imagine them knowing, like wise tribal elders. We hug a lot, and I clutch my son's photo against my chest, the image facing outward, so that people who really want to see it can see it, and people who prefer not to look at dead babies can avert their eyes.

Kevin and I clasp our hands together and turn to walk over the tracks, down the steps, and out onto the beach, not really knowing where we're going. People take this cue to follow us. I kick off my sandals, cold shards of seashell sticking to the bottoms of my bare feet, and find strange comfort in this mildly painful sensation. As I propel myself forward like a robot, tears free-fall down my face, warm and salty, traveling all the way down my neckline.

"Shit, Kleenex," says Kevin. "I knew we forgot something."

It's what he knows, what he can do: taking care of those sorts of details. Releasing his hand from mine, he rummages in his pocket for something Kleenex-like, but comes up empty.

"It's fide," I say, my nose completely clogged. "Who deeds Kleedex. That's what farmer's blows are for."

I try to smile, but I can't. Just plain can't, because the puppety, roboty feeling is dissipating, and I now feel ravaged and stinging. Everything just sucks and hurts. Kevin takes my hand again, and we stop at a patch of sand close to where the icy waves are lapping up at our feet, turning away from the water to face the small crowd that has begun to gather tightly around us in a crescent shape. Paul and my mom stand beside us as we face the crowd, with the loud, slate-gray ocean as our backdrop.

We all take out our respective crumpled sheets of paper, scrawled with what we have planned to say. Mine is typed. The rain has dwindled to a mere sprinkling of fine drops, thank God. Paul goes first, and then Mom.

Their speeches are filled with lovey, supporty, community-esque things, both remarking at how great it is to have everyone come together like this. Then there is mine, rambling and repetitive and filled with all sorts of clichés.

And finally, there is Kevin, whose speech is the most concise and show-stopping of all, its poignant meaning perfectly carved out in just a few, artfully chosen words. He says it quietly, tears just behind his eyes, hard emotion just beneath the surface:

*Dear Son,*

*Forgive me when I cry. It's certainly not what I would have taught you to do. Occasionally, I can't help it. I can't help it when I see your mother's face fill with pain. I can't help it when I replay her phone call in my head. "There's something wrong with the baby," she said. I can't help it when times that were supposed to be so joyous are filled with crushing disappointment —the day of your baby shower, your due date, the three months of paternity leave that we would have spent together, all the baseball games that we would have watched and played. Forgive me when I cry, and know that I'll never forget the seven and a half months of joy you brought to us.*

*Dear Son,*

*Forgive me for the times that I don't cry. Most of the time, I can't help but be happy, and it's hard not to feel guilty about that. I can't help but be happy when your mother dances in the living room. I can't help it when family and friends visit and bring us food, prop us up with support, watch football and play ping-pong with us. I can't help but be happy that I'm married to your mother and knowing that we'll make it, stay positive, and have more kids in the near future. I can't help being happy because it's my nature, and your mother brings it out in me, as she does in everyone else. Forgive me when I don't cry, and know that I'll never forget the seven and a half months of joy you brought to us.*

*Love, Dad*

His speech leaves everyone breathless and silent, frozen and watching him. I stare back down at my white, bare feet, numb with coldness, because I can't bear to look up at his profile beside me, his lower lip trembling.

After everyone has spoken, Kevin nods in my direction, and we both turn to face the water. I hike my skirt up to my knees, follow him out

147

until we are calf-deep, and balance myself precariously between slimy, barnacle-covered rocks beneath the surface. Kevin pulls a small white box from his pocket, and from that a clear plastic bag filled with gray dust, and he pours half of the dust into my hand, and the other half into his. It seems strangely meaningless, surreal, holding this tiny cloud of nothingness and doing something supposedly useful with it. Who's to say that these are really the ashes of my child, or ashes at all? And why are we throwing them into the ocean?

I don't know, truthfully, but we do it anyway, mechanically, ritualistically. Just as I imagined, throwing dust isn't easy, especially on a breezy, drizzly day at the beach. I clumsily attempt to toss my handful outward toward the sea as my hair blows into my mouth. The dust blows every which way as I open my hand, back against my white cardigan sweater and some of it still stuck to my palm, which I brush off with my other palm, winding up with a thin ashen coating on both hands. This is just weird. I finally bend down and submerge both hands in the icy water, rubbing them together. I guess that'll work. With waves hitting my knees, I turn and stumble back to shore. Kevin follows at my heels.

Nina is the person whose eyes meet mine first, and she steps forward, arms extended. Her expression is wide open and steeped in sorrow, corners of her mouth turned downward. I practically fall against her and we embrace for a long time, connected, while everybody else hugs everybody else and the salty wind blows around us. She knows how absurdly, maddeningly sad and stupid all of this is. It's the first time we've really ever hugged in such a long, hard, real way, and it feels strangely like a goodbye. *Goodbye, friend. Our roads are parting. Catch you on the flip side.* My face on her shoulder, I squeeze my eyes shut, tears seeping out anyway.

I guess that's what this whole morning is supposed to be all about: saying goodbye to a piece of life.

# The Fourth Journey Segment:
## From an Uncharted, Upward-Seeming Path to Somewhere
*October to December, 2007*

## In Search of Fresh Victims

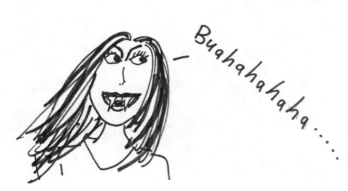

Buahahahaha.....

WHEN YOUR BABY'S ASHES are doing whatever things do when they get dumped into the ocean, I suppose one would expect a bit of subsequent relief. Some closure, a release from the shackles of strangeness and melancholy, a newfound ability to move on. What's the point of a funeral, of making someone's ashes disappear forever, if not that? Not that I regret the memorial, but it somehow isn't making me feel as liberated from loss as I'd hoped. Perhaps that's because I'm more aware of that loss than ever, acutely sensing its thick, tar-like presence just underneath my skin.

I'm alone in my shared office at the college. The building feels empty, most instructors having already left in a scramble to beat traffic. A single bird is chirping in the courtyard. This past week I've become overwhelmed by unread e-mail messages and ungraded essays piling up, several weeks of classes that have yet to be planned, and the growing film of grime and sticky sweet coffee rings on my desktop. I feel behind in everything, trapped in a permanent state of disorganization, like a scatterbrained cockroach living underneath a jumbled heap of rubbish.

I start to feel sorry as I push papers halfheartedly around my desk—not sorry for myself, which seems to be the most recent norm—but sorry for Zachary, for attempting to replace him so quickly with various things. Parties, adoption fairs, this new job. What have I really done to acknowledge his existence, or show others that I still want to talk about him? The funeral counts for something, I suppose, but that only lasted about thirty minutes—not a very big proportion of the total time he's been gone. There are probably some other times too that I'm not thinking of now, like the blue announcements with the dragonfly design. But it seems that for the most part, I've allowed him to be ignored because dead babies are like the ultimate short-bus kid – the oddball that nobody wants to mention.

I am overcome with the sudden urge to forcibly share my baby with at least one coworker, to show the world that just because he is dead doesn't mean he is less cute than any other baby. And if I ruffle a few feathers in the process, make my innocent victims uncomfortable as they get dragged down into Monica's black stillbirth world, so be it.

Impulsively, I open up some electronic photos of Zachary that the nurses took, and that have been saved in my e-mail for months: a close-up of his profile and one of his chubby feet. I decide to post them online with a slate-colored background and little captions for each picture, for this seems like a safe starting point for sharing my infant son more openly and proudly. I'm fairly certain the pre-knocked-down me wouldn't have condoned posting macabre photographs of dead bodies online, particularly while I'm at work, where I doubt I'm getting paid to do such non-academic things. But I can't help myself, and—feeling as though I'm doing something dangerous and naughty like perusing Internet porn, I turn my computer screen slightly away from my office door. Then, figuring I may as well start at the top, I pound out an e-mail message to Audrey, the Arts and Humanities chair, and attach a link to the gallery site. I tell her that I wanted to share these with someone—I hope she doesn't find them gruesome—and that I totally understand if she'd prefer not to see them. Content with this concise and purposeful message, I click "send."

Next, I gaze out the partially open sliding-glass doors of my office into the sunlit courtyard, contemplating who my next forced-informing victim will be. A few doors down, I hear some rustling sounds, and the upbeat voice of a woman talking on the phone. It's Shelly, an older instructor who happens to be one of the nicest, most well loved people in the whole building. She's the kind of person who smiles and laughs a lot, and wears artsy clothing—bold colors and big, jingly-jangly jewelry that probably comes from street fairs. Because of that, and because she happens to be here at this precise moment, I decide that she's the one. Fresh blood. I stand up and step outside, only to practically bump head-on into Shelly herself.

"Oh hi, Monica!" she says.

"Hey, Shelly." I pause for a moment, shuffling around on my feet. "Um, I was just wondering if…I could show you something. It'll only take a second."

"Sure!" She follows me into my office. Such a nice person, she is. Wiggling the computer mouse around and opening up Zachary's profile shot, I feel momentarily bad for roping her into my world of death.

"I just want to show you a picture of my son Zachary," I say carefully, nervously. "I mean, I know he's dead and all. But nobody here has ever seen him before, and I don't want people to be…like…afraid of him like he's some kind of zombie-baby freak."

Shelly leans in to get a closer look. "Wow. He's a beautiful boy," she says softly, her smile fading a tiny bit.

"Really?" I say, proud of my child, maybe for the very first time ever, proud to brag about him like mommies of normal babies do. It feels like I just lost a lot of weight, and now I get to parade around in those size-four jeans that I could never wear before. I'm being a new mom. "I think he's pretty cute myself. Look at his little nose. Those dark spots on his face are from dead skin, they told me. Otherwise, he's perfect. Just over six pounds. Oh, and check this one out."

I open the other picture, this one of his two pudgy feet poking out from underneath a flannel blanket, each with five tiny toes. They look just like the feet of a real baby.

"He's a handsome one," Shelly whispers, gazing at the photographs for a long time, her earrings jingle-jangling together, glinting in the light.

"Yeah, I know," I say, relieved that this conversation isn't as torturous as I thought it might be.

She looks up from the computer screen. "You know, Monica, I think it's great you keep these photos of Zachary, and I'm so honored to get to see them. I had a miscarriage once, a long time ago. Sometimes I wish I'd taken more time to say goodbye to that baby. Just, you know, feel something toward it. But I didn't. I just went on with my life without looking back. There are still days when I regret it."

"Really?"

"Yeah. So, you're doing a good thing here, Monica."

We exchange a long, quiet hug, and I feel as though I'm hovering in a moment of pure, human connection. Pleased that someone from the work compartment of my life has now seen my baby, and not only didn't run away screaming in horror, but divulged to me a similar experience from her own life. After she leaves, I look back down at my desk, which is still in abysmal shape, and decide it's too late in the day to get anything else done. I write "STAY LATE TODAY TO GET ORGANIZED" on a sticky note and affix it to my computer monitor in a place where I'll see it tomorrow, and head out into the sun-drenched parking lot where my car is sloppily parked at a slight angle.

The traffic is predictably bad on my drive home, but it doesn't bother me as much as usual. I shared a piece of myself today. I hope Zachary witnessed the whole thing from wherever dead people go—even if he's embarrassed that his mother is going around sharing his naked-baby photos.

*It's a part of life*, I tell him. *Mom gets to show you off.*

## Family Involvement

HERE'S THE AGGRAVATING THING about explanations. There's no shortage of them when you're worried about something that's probably nothing, like a slow-moving baby. On the other hand, when it's something that really is something—like a *dead* baby—they're nowhere to be found. Where are they when I need them the most, those elusive, formerly abundant explanations? So many questions, none with answers.

What caused the surface of our baby's heart to calcify like an eggshell? Could it have been prevented? Detected earlier, perhaps? Could it happen again? Was the first miscarriage related to this? Believe me, I would love to know something, to know what danger to look for in the future, what to avoid. The problem is that the doctors themselves don't know—they've already admitted to that. And no matter how many variations of the words "stillbirth," "fetal," "heart calcification," "causes," and "what the fuck happened" I type into Google, staring searchingly at the blue-white glow of my computer screen, nothing comes up.

My mom is searching too; I can feel it. Whenever she calls, our conversations are smattered with her probing questions disguised as innocent musings: "Honey, I read online that it could be caused by a recessive gene…" Then her voice trails off as she waits for me to jump in with some revolutionary piece of information that I discovered since our last phone call. I tell her if I had a juicy response to give her, I would. But I never do, and such discussions only leave me feeling inexplicably irritated and frustrated, wondering why Mom won't accept that there *aren't any answers*, wishing my own thought patterns weren't so similar to hers beneath the surface. Irritation then melts into guilt, for this is hardly the

154

time to revert back to that petulant thirteen-year-old-version of myself, always annoyed with my mom. Kevin's mom asks him lots of questions too, but he doesn't get irritated.

Anyway, who's to blame our mothers for asking, for attempting to make sense of this nameless, faceless misfortune that has hurt and shocked our entire family? Instinct is to protect us all. To pinpoint the cause, take measures to prevent recurrence, and move forward. Kevin and our dads seem better at accepting the mysterious, random cruelty of nature. Must be a guy-thing. One of these days, we females might learn to live with not understanding. We might all become more Zen-like, wise enough to know and accept what we can't control.

OUT OF THE BLUE, I get a call from my dad in St. Louis. He never just phones on his own; usually it's Mom who initiates random calls, with Dad listening in.

"Are you around this weekend?" he says. "I thought I'd come up for a visit."

My heart skips a beat because this is so unprecedented. "Really? This coming weekend? Just like...by yourself? What's Mom up to?"

"Well, she was just up there for the funeral, you know, so she thought she'd just stick around St. Louis."

"That would be awesome! Yeah, I'll be around."

Wow; a spontaneous father-daughter visit! This hasn't happened since I don't know when. That Friday evening, a yellow cab pulls up in on the shoulder of the road in front of our house. Through the foggy darkness, I see my dad's familiar form—medium height, slight shoulders, brown jacket, beat-up leather shoulder bag that used to be my grandfather's. As I walk out onto the damp front porch in my bare feet, then down the cold concrete steps toward him, I can make out his face in the yellow streetlight, Irish and angular, ever so slightly gaunt in the cheeks. His dark brown hair is turning silver in places. He looks up and smiles in my direction.

"Sorry I'm late," he says, his smile fading just a tiny bit. I know he means late for the memorial service.

"It's okay. Here, let me carry that. How was your flight?" I grab his shoulder bag with one hand, and wrap my other arm around his waist as we walk up the front steps together.

"Oh, fine. You know, the usual."

When we get into the warm house, he takes off his shoes and tosses his coat on the futon, and I set his leather bag down on the floor in the office-formerly-known-as-baby-room.

"We can bring the futon mattress in here later, okay, Dad?" I say, returning to the living room. "That way you can have some privacy. Have you eaten yet?"

Now that his coat is off, I can see he's wearing my favorite cream-colored, cable knit wool sweater from Ireland. He's had it for as long as I can remember. I've seen pictures of myself in his arms as a toddler, my head resting on his shoulder, him in that same wool sweater. Suddenly, I'm flooded with an unidentifiable emotion, a big ball of love and hurt and sadness, longing for the past, for innocent dreams and babies, lost.

I throw my arms around his neck and lean against him limply, burying my face in his scratchy wool sweater and crying with quiet force. He smells like Dad, like salt and Dial soap and Gillette shaving cream. This makes me cry harder. Without a word, he strokes the back of my head with one hand and holds me against him with the other, and I feel small and young, like a child again. We stand like that for several frozen minutes until his wool-clad shoulder is soaked, and I pull back, feeling the redness and swollenness of my eyes.

"I'm so sorry this happened to you," he says, looking straight at me, his expression open and solemn. "I didn't realize until you sent those pictures that he was...a real baby. I just...wish you didn't have to go through this. I can't imagine."

We lock gazes for several seconds as he shakes his head sorrowfully.

"S'okay, Dad. I deed a Kleedex."

With that oh-so-attractive stuffed nose voice, I run into the kitchen to grab a paper towel, blowing so hard that I just about cause my eardrums to burst. On the way back, I grab Zach's framed photos off the dining room table—the one of his feet and the other of his profile.

"These are the pictures the durses took," I say. "You already saw them—I bead, they're the sabe ones I e-bailed you."

We sit down on the area rug, and Dad studies each picture closely, shaking his head again.

"What a shame," he says, and I feel myself swell with pride and relief. *Grandpa knows you now*, I think upward, toward Zachary.

Dad, Kevin and I spend the weekend doing not much of anything— just taking long walks and having drawn-out conversations, sometimes about the baby and sometimes not. We talk about dad-stuff: our basement and finances, the Iraq War, my brother's life as a perpetual bachelor. We take naps and go out for greasy junk-food dinners. It reminds me of when my mom used to go out of town on business trips, and Dad would take Paul and me to McDonald's or Kentucky Fried Chicken for dinner. Something about my dad's presence makes me feel serene and safe. Yet another point lost by the grief literature, which never mentioned a damn thing about the healing powers of just hanging out with your dad.

157

# A MILD TANTRUM

I'M RATHER ENJOYING THIS KICK of showing Zachary to the world, like he's part of a slide show from my most recent overseas vacation. *Every*one should see him and his big, lifeless profile! We ought to host a movie night in our living room with friends, showing Zach's photographs—all two of them—with Kevin and me narrating in the background. It would be like a dead-baby-baby-shower, all about that baby and me: our moment in the sun. How could anybody not love that?

The next show-and-tell opportunity comes with a visit from Kevin's parents—Jim and Kate—and his younger brother Brian. They've decided to fly up from San Diego for a few days. I've always enjoyed conversations with Kevin's family: deeper than superficial, yet coasting cheerily and safely above topics that might be uncomfortably touchy, that might acknowledge any kind of personal awfulness a bit too explicitly.

Now, though, I find myself harboring a secret hope that this year's visit will be an exception, even though the matter of Zachary surely falls outside the conversational comfort zone of the LeMoine family. It's all a part of my quest for public acknowledgement of my dead kid. Before they show up, I get our son's story ready to tell, compiling all of his peripheral relics on the roll top desk in the office. The charred metal disc etched with his crematorium ID number, the plastic baggie with remnants of his ashes, the black and white photographs in wooden frames.

The family arrives, Brian sleeping on our futon in the basement, Kate and Jim checking into a nearby hotel with their Marriott Rewards points. We do typical family things – happy hours in the living room with Hickory Farms cheese and sausage, trips to Pike Place Market, dinners of pork roasts and mashed potatoes, drawn out discussions about the woes in Iraq and the latest fiber news on the cover of *Nutrition Action*. All the while, I wait patiently, eagerly, for a clear segue, an opportunity to show everyone the artifacts of my pregnancy, my son, my loss. Waiting for someone to say, *Tell us about the baby! What it was like to deliver! Do you have any other baby pictures to share?* so that I can reply, *Why yes! Funny you should ask! I just happen to have a complete exhibit set up in the office at this very moment. It's called Zachary: Les Objets de Sa Vie. Let's go into the office now and I'll give you a tour!*

But by the last night of their visit, none of these things has come up, and the little Zachary-museum that I meticulously assembled has gone unseen. I feel myself turning into a big, wound-up ball of sulkiness, feigning brittle cheerfulness on the outside. I know their actions aren't intentional, that I ought to relax. But it's much easier to sit here grumpily and fume about it.

We all walk down to the pizzeria on 5th Avenue for our final family dinner, crowding around a table with a red-checkered cloth. The discussion revolves around Grandma LeMoine's eightieth birthday surprise party being planned by all of her kids. I find myself bothered by the fact that Grandma's birthday party should get to take up the entire conversational spotlight at dinner, while the biggest, baddest event of the year—the one thing occupying eighty percent of my brain day after day, and clearly the more important topic—doesn't even get a two-second honorable mention. Tuning in and out, I chew petulantly on a slice of pepperoni pizza, the lights starting to seem too bright and my throat getting dry.

"...and then you and Monica can make a big sign that says 'Happy Birthday Grandma,' and—"

Pushing abruptly back from the table, I stand up and rush toward the front door, weaving through people and chairs and pizza-laden tables, stepping out into the chilly dark night. There, I find a little nook in the brick wall of the building and wedge myself into it, folding my arms across my chest. My first temper tantrum in front of the in-laws: how embarrassing. Seconds later, Kevin appears.

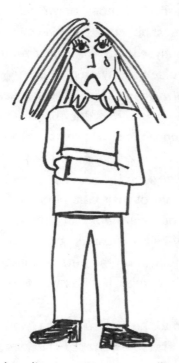

"Here," he says, handing me my coat, pulling me toward him as I shove my arms through the sleeves. "It's not because they don't care."

"Okay but…why are they afraid to, like, even mention it?" I blubber woefully into his shoulder, my voice muffled and snotty.

"They don't know what to say. It's awkward for people, and plus they have no idea that you're dying to talk about it. That's just the way it is."

"Why? Why the fuck is it awkward?" My voice rises in pitch like a whiny (and foul-mouthed) child. "Can't they bring it up just once? Can't they just…predict what I want without me having to beg for it? Just a simple 'how've you been doing since the baby died?' Same with our friends, for that matter. Nina and Carrie and Jane are the only ones who haven't basically disappeared off the planet, in case you haven't noticed. Don't I get, like, a celebration or a dead-baby shower or something? Is it 'cuz he was stillborn? So that makes him like this fucking diseased mutant alien child? Why don't people—"

I stop and breathe in sharply, feeling suddenly as though it isn't really me talking anymore, but some scary, hypersensitive version of myself that I'd rather not get to know. A big old cry-baby; that's what I am. The grief experts would tell me to do the mature and proactive thing: just tell people outright that hey, I need to talk about Zachary for a while. That's all. It wouldn't be so hard. People would at least know what I needed, and they would probably listen politely—even empathetically—just like Shelly did.

The door beside us creaks open, and a warm waft of pizza-scented air drifts out.

"Are you all right?" It's Kate's voice.

I jerk my head up from Kevin's shoulder, sniffling. "Yeah, I'm fine. Sorry."

"Well Monica, it's just awful, what you've been through. We all wish we could make it better."

"Thanks."

Brian and Jim trail out next, Jim mumbling something about how this place always ends up being more expensive than you think it's going to be, which is true. We walk home in the frigid darkness, Kevin and me lagging behind the others, his arm slung over my shoulder. I'm shocked, still, that he continues to feel any affection toward me at all. The discussion is a flurry of travel logistics now—what time people's flights leave tomorrow, where to return the rental car. I stare down at the black sidewalk lines moving past, attempting to step on each one, achingly regretful about having melted down in front of Kevin's perfectly nice parents and brother. I've now probably pushed them away forever, dashing any future hope that they might broach the topic I want so desperately to talk about. *Good thing we never brought up the baby,* they're probably thinking. *She can't even handle going out for pizza.*

"I'm sorry," I say to Kevin that night as we're washing dishes. Brian is downstairs watching TV.

"Sorry about what?" He hands me a clean, dripping plate to add to the drying rack, and turns off the faucet.

"You know. Sorry for acting stupid."

"You weren't acting stupid. We gotta just…keep things in perspective."

Just then, the phone rings. I wipe my hands on the front of my sweatshirt and pick it up. It's Mindy—Kevin's other brother's wife, calling from Los Angeles. Mindy, with two babies of her own, has been more vocally and dramatically upset about the stillbirth than anyone in either of our families. She was a theatre major; maybe that's why.

"Hey—Rob and I just called to say hi. I know the family is there and all—sorry we couldn't make it up to Seattle. How're you guys doing?"

"All right," I say.

"Hey, I know it doesn't come up much in conversation, but I wanted you to know that everyone in the family is thinking about you and the baby. It doesn't show much, but it affected all of us. Rob cried for a few hours the night it happened. We talk about it a lot, just not when you're around. Nobody wants to upset you."

"Really?"

"Yeah. We're all just…so relieved that you and Kevin made it through in one piece. We're rooting for you."

"Thanks, Mindy. That means a lot. Wanna talk to Kev?"

"Sure, I'll say hi."

I hand the phone over and notice—for the first time in weeks—the lush, green plant that Kate and Jim sent us after the baby died. It's displayed on the fireplace mantel, flowy philodendron tendrils mixed with other unknown foliage, spilling out of a pretty woven basket. This one outlasted all of the extravagant flower arrangements and multi-layered casseroles we received, and continues to thrive in its own strong and understated way, blending right into the other plants and candles and photographs in the living room. Right then, I decide that this must be how Kevin's family is there for us: subtly, constantly, like soothing background noise.

Probably a bullshit analogy, but I'm proud of myself for thinking of it nonetheless.

# A Tea Party Gone Awry

I COULD REALLY USE A DOSE OF RAUNCHY, gossipy, wine-spiked girl talk. So I decide to organize a booze-and-estrogen fest under the guise of a "tea party." Thursday afternoon seems best, for that's when the Baby Ladies are most available. I know I already issued an unspoken "goodbye" to them at the memorial service, a farewell to the life they represent, but in truth I find myself still clinging to those relationshps like they're some kind of drug. The goal right now is to hang out with girlfriends, not babies, even though I know that the presence of babies is inevitable.

I'm okay with that, because—for the most part—I think I'm over the whole "woe is me, I'm feeling a little piqued at the sight of your baby" thing. Besides, surely the babies will fall asleep in the next room, sit quietly and not make any noise, or—better yet—be left at home altogether with a neighbor or a husband. Surely, the conversation will focus not on babies, but on more exciting adult subject matter, such as the hotness of the latest male movie star. As an added psychological safety net, I've also added "DOGS WELCOME" to the invite, figuring that a whirlwind of romping pups in the house might be a pleasant detractor from baby centeredness. It will be like the babies aren't even there.

So here I am on the day of, buzzed from a super-size mug of afternoon coffee. I've put together some mini Greek chicken wraps from scratch, bound them with toothpicks for an extra fancy touch, and arranged them in concentric patterns on plates. Several bottles of Sutter Home white zinfandel are chilling in the fridge, and I've popped in a swing music CD to liven up the atmosphere. Not that any "livening" will be needed here, thank you very much. These are my *home*girls, and talking shit is what we *do*! Sunlight streams through the window and onto the glass coffee table, highlighting my fine Windexing abilities. I am feeling Martha Stewart cool and on top of my game.

My kid-free friend Marcie, along with her big basset hound and cousin Pam, are the first to show up. Jane, Carrie and Nina then arrive one by one, along with their massive entourages of babies, baby carriers, and bags of baby gear. Everyone has also brought a container of homemade cookies to share with the exception of Nina, who has little Damon in one arm and an enormous, half-full bottle of Jack Daniels wedged in the opposite armpit. Rover, her little black dog that was the precursor to Damon, trots in behind her.

"Leftover from the wedding," she says, grinning as she sets the bottle down on our countertop. It doesn't slip by unnoticed, this subtle reminder that Nina doesn't drink that kind of stuff anymore, at least not for now (but I certainly can, and do), that we've gone from best prego buddies to living on totally different planets. Ouch. I feel a pinch of sadness, barely a pinprick. Thankfully, it passes quickly.

The living room fills with loud, sing-songy hellos and boisterous hugs.

"Hiiiiiii! Haven't seen you in SO long!"

"Oh my goodness, look how *big* he's getting!"

The first few minutes are consumed by the mommies unpacking their babies and baggage, spreading out with binkies and bottles and what nots, and oohing and ahhing over each other's offspring, who are now unstrapped from their carriers and lying all over living room floor. Meanwhile, I mill about the room, giving hugs and making general announcements about how cute and chubby all the infants look.

When it becomes apparent that babies and dogs don't mix well in such a small space, we all agree that the dogs—and not the babies—will have to be relegated to the backyard. I'm mildly disappointed—but not surprised—by this group decision.

Bustling back and forth between the kitchen and living room, arranging cookies on plates and heating up water for tea, I debate about whether or not to crack open a bottle of wine. I've announced that it's there, but nobody's expressed any interest. The second disappointing glitch of the afternoon. But then again, what on earth was I expecting? For these dutiful new mothers to drive home drunk with their infants in the back seat? I decide on a mug of Earl Gray instead; no need to be the lone, red-faced wino in the room, you know.

I then settle in beside Pam, who is sitting stoically on the futon. Marcie is bubbly as ever, going from baby to baby to coo and take pictures. Jane's corner of the room already looks like a veritable kiddie-food laboratory, lined with plastic containers of pureed yams and peas and other this-and-that's, a veritable buffet of organic nutrition for baby Jeffrey, who is the oldest child present. The room is abuzz with chatter about sleeping and feeding and skin rashes. I initiate small talk with Pam, asking her what her husband does, what her dog is like, why she decided to go to nursing school. Our conversation fizzles within a few minutes, however, and we both turn our attention to the mommies sitting around on the floor.

By this point, I've come down from my earlier caffeine high. Sorry, but Earl Gray just doesn't cut it; I've always been suspicious of people who claim to get high from drinking tea. I begin to feel ever so slightly adrift, disconcerted, like an outsider at my own party. I can't seem to get into a good conversational groove with any of the Baby Ladies on the floor, for I've no insightful tips to offer, no ability to commiserate with their breast feeding woes or sleepless nights. I can't relate to the single thing that is dominating all three of their lives right now—new motherhood—nor do I have the capacity to smother their babies with the affection and attention they surely deserve and are used to. I attempt to break into a few conversations from my position atop the futon, making occasional bitchy comments about suburbia and Paris Hilton, hoping to spark some juicier discussion, but it all keeps coming back to babies. Babies, babies, babies. Motherfucking babies.

I grab one of Carrie's espresso shortbread biscuits and pop the entire thing into my mouth, chewing slowly and gazing over the wiggly babies and mommies' heads and out the window at the great dense pine tree in front of our house. In a brief moment of shining clarity, I become acutely aware of the truth—the in-your-face, can't-deny-it truth: the topic of babies, and, indeed, the babies themselves, still causes me so much distress that I am literally afraid to touch or look too closely at any of the adorable infants writhing around on the floor. I am decidedly not "over babies" as I thought I would be by now, and wonder if I ever will be. What's worse, the sense of camaraderie I once felt with Nina and Carrie and Jane simply no longer exists. That's how this feels, anyway. I'm the odd man out, the one who didn't get invited to the party that everyone's raving about, the girl who didn't even get a bit part in the school play that everyone else is in.

As I return from being lost in negative thought, a ray of bright sunlight shines directly on my face, and the room feels hot and stuffy. Damn, this house is small. How much did we pay for it? I am irritated by the sun, by the Seattle real estate market, by this boring mug of tea. How unfair and cruel of me, I think, to put so many innocent babies and new mommies in the position of being in the same room as an old scrooge like me, someone who is literally pained by their collective presence. I utter a quick mental prayer to the great being above, the one who isn't listening anyway: *Please, whoever's up there: let these babies and mommies not be tainted in any way by my negative aura.*

"I'll be right back," I say with forced cheerfulness, and proceed to busy myself again with important hostess responsibilities, like adjusting the music volume and replenishing the food supply. Pam and Marcie both make their way into the kitchen, and the three of us start our own side conversation, completely separate from the mommies in the living room. A little subgroup of childless women; that's us. I meander outside intermittently to check on the dogs, even though there's not much to check on. Rover is staring desperately through the crack in the door, telepathically begging Nina to rescue him from this strange yard and strange dog who isn't his friend.

During a lull in the discussion, I decide to put a dent in the dishes piling up in the sink, and Nina appears beside me. My arms are immersed in warm soapy water, and we chat for a few minutes. Small talk, mostly.

We ask each other about our respective husbands, I ask her how the house hunt is going. Our conversation seems stunted and strained to me, and I feel myself again becoming acutely, painfully aware of the chasm between my life and hers.

"Uh, so…I overheard you saying Damon's sleeping better these days?" I say. Her child. What else is there to talk about, really.

"Yeah, he's doing okay. I'm still really shocked by all of his sleeping problems—I never expected any of it, you know? I mean, I was so set on just getting through the delivery that I really wasn't thinking beyond that."

Her words are airy and staccato, light and good-natured the way Nina's words usually are. I've always loved the ease of our conversations. But to me, right now, they feel like a kick in the stomach. I swallow hard, grab the greasiest pan within reach, and begin scrubbing it like a housewife on speed.

"Mmmm," I respond. "So, are you…um…going back to work this year?"

"Well, I don't think so. I think we're gonna try to have a second baby soon, you know, just to get both of 'em out of the way up front, and then I can start back to work in like four years or something."

Kick in the stomach number two. I scrub harder. Poor Nina is the innocent party in all of this, for she is not at fault for my current, hypersensitive state of mind. Nor is she to blame for that fact that I, masochist that I am, insist on asking these mommies questions about their babies, even knowing their answers will feel like rubbing alcohol being poured into my own cuts.

What I want most of all is to feel normal. Balanced. Low-maintenance. Strong. Dignified. I thought I was making progress in that direction, wasn't I? I want to maintain my Martha Stewart image, calm and collected under pressure. Why is it so fucking hard to ask my friend, my good friend, a simple question about her life? I long for a replenishment of positive energy so that I can channel it out and suck it back in, but all I'm coming up with are dark, pissy, sad feelings. I fling greasy water off my hands, say something like "mmmm" again, and go back out into the living room.

The culminating moment of the afternoon happens shortly thereafter, when another kid-free friend, Callie, comes bursting in the back door nearly an hour late with her gigantic dog Tang behind her. The other pups sneak in through the open door, and all three dogs come galloping ecstatically into the cramped living room like a tornado of high-velocity tails and tongues and legs, causing mass chaos to ensue.

"WATCH THE BABIES!!" Nina shouts frantically. On instinct, the mommies shield the children from stomping dog paws and snatch up open containers of food, as Tang's powerfully wagging tail whacks everything in sight.

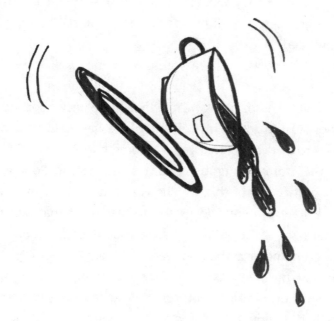

"WATCH THE IKEA RUG!" I shout, equally frantically. Mugs and glasses and cookies and half-eaten chicken wraps go flying off the coffee table, directly onto—yes—the rug. The room has become like a Baghdad battle zone, a spinning tornado of waving arms, wagging tails, fluffy little dogs, distraught mommy-faces, flying food, and streams of tepid liquid. Lizzie, the basset hound, seizes the moment—grabbing a whole chicken wrap off the floor and disappearing into the kitchen. I'm on my hands and knees, gingerly picking up crumbs and food scraps that have fallen. The flying vectors of tea have already formed puddles on the hardwood floor and the coffee tabletop.

"Oh my God, I'm so sorry!" says Callie, joining the general scramble to get the dogs back outside. I follow her in that direction to gather paper towels, passing Lizzie, who is hunkering in the corner of the kitchen, scarfing down her big score of the afternoon.

Everyone laughs nervously once the situation is back under control, the messes cleaned up, dogs safely shut outdoors. There are attempts to resume normal conversation, but the convivial mood has been stymied to the point of no return. Five minutes later, Jane stands up abruptly and says, "Well, we gotta get going. Thanks for a great time!"

And that is, much to my relief, the impetus for everyone else to get going too.

Alone in the house again, I sink down into the orange futon, the same futon on which baby Zachary was originally conceived, and the male fetus before him. Billy Holiday sings softly in the background, and tears spill out of my eyes and run down my chin. I sniffle and snort, attempting to swallow back my snot because I'm too lazy to grab a tissue from the bathroom.

I have another sudden flashback to my younger days, this time of something my mom said when I was seventeen. I had just been dumped by my first real boyfriend, Carl, with whom I had lost my virginity, gotten high, and skipped school for the first time. Important adolescent milestones, indeed. Many a starry summer night we had spent lying in the grass, talking excitedly and semi-seriously about getting married, and plotting ways to escape school together. I went away for the summer to volunteer in Idaho, and things were inexplicably different between us when I came back. When Carl and I were sitting barefoot on his front porch and he suggested that we "cool it" for a while, I was about as hurt as a seventeen-year-old can be from such a thing. For about a month thereafter, I took to calling him every few days, sticking notes in his locker, and spending extra time teasing my bangs in hopes of rekindling his attraction to me. We even attempted to make out a few more times in the backseat of his car, parked behind Denny's, but the connection was clearly gone. Finally, my mom pulled me aside .

"Honey, you're not with him anymore," she said. "You've got to move on and stop calling him. You're smart and beautiful, and you'll get through this. Let's go see *Aladdin*."

At the time, I was annoyed and insulted by her unsolicited advice and her suggestion that I go out in public with my parents to see a cartoon flick, even though *Aladdin* turned out not to be a half-bad movie. But now, fifteen years later, the brilliance of her advice suddenly resonates. Those heady, pregnant days with my baby lady friends are over, the things we used to talk about no longer valid, the common excitement—that glass snow-globe world I was living in—gone. Had it, lost it, won't get it back. I remember one of the many grief pamphlet shoved into my arms listing "acceptance" as a stage of grief and I wonder briefly if this is it, if this is what "acceptance" means.

It means it's time for me to let go of more than half of my closest girlfriends in this rainy-ass city, even though it's about the hardest thing I can imagine. Time to do what I think I've known for a while, deep down in some part of my heart that I preferred to ignore: let go of that old world, and make a new one for myself.

Or, as Mom would say: *time to move on.*

# SLOPPY SECONDS

"KEV, CAN WE GET A PARROT?"

I suppose some might view parrot-motherhood as sloppy seconds, begrudgingly embraced by people who can't produce real offspring. Still, these past few weeks I've decided that having a small, warm creature to nurture (tiny enough, even, to fit inside my belly if he or she were curled up just right) would be a welcome new focal point, and part of my "acceptance" path. Part of moving on, as Mom would call it. And I don't need Nina or Carrie or anybody else to help me do it.

"We've already talked about this," Kevin reminds me. "I don't want a loud, obnoxious bird shitting all over our furniture. Besides, we're both allergic and we travel too much."

"But parrots are hypoallergenic, I swear. We can leave him at a bird daycare or something when we go away. Oh, and I'm pretty sure you can get bird-diapers online."

"That's stupid. I don't want a parrot."

"But—"

"We're not getting a parrot."

I've asked too soon—entirely a misjudgment on my part. The trick to getting a "yes" out of Kevin is to appeal to his sense of practicality; that is, to do the necessary research first, and return with a more informed approach. Racing back into the office, I print out enormous quantities of information on parrots' dietary and emotional needs, stuffing it into what used to be called the "Adoption Info" folder. I've ceremoniously crossed those out the word "Adoption," writing "Parrot" above it in black marker. Visions of life with our new parrot-child unfold easily in my mind. With

Kevin's assistance, I'll build a gigantic aviary of chicken wire in the back yard, where our parrot can live in the summer months. Ours will be fed nothing but the best quality vegetables and grains, and sit on a specially built bath-ledge while I shower so that he can bask in a warm waterfall alongside me, happily preening in the misty air. It will be as though he never left the rainforest.

I bring up the subject with Kevin a few days later, this time armed with my now-bulging "Parrot Info" folder, but he gives me the "no way in hell" look again.

Damn. Time to shift my focus away from birds.

I sift through my mental log of other pet possibilities that might be more palatable to Kevin. Dogs and cats—especially cats—are most likely out of the question, because they make us both sneeze. Reptiles and fish are about the most depressing pets one could possibly have, for they do nothing but hover behind glass with vapid expressions. Hamsters and gerbils are no better. A potbellied pig, maybe.

"I'd consider a dog," Kevin finally calls into the office, where I'm busy writing down names and numbers of potbellied pig dealers. I set down my pen and go sit beside him on the futon.

"Really? A dog? But, what about allergies?"

"Poodle mixes are supposed to be okay for that. I don't want to come home from work one day and find a parrot or a pig in the house, which I know is where you're headed. If that's what it comes down to, I'd rather have a dog." That's my man: king of damage control.

"I wouldn't just go out and buy a parrot or a pig without your knowledge," I say.

"Yeah you would, especially when you're in one of your...obsessed moods."

He's right. I realize, with jubilant satisfaction, that I have gotten Kevin to agree to getting a pet—maybe not a parrot, but a pet nonetheless—by forcing him to choose between something already illogical (like a dog) and something even less logical (like a parrot or a pig). It seems that I've generated so much mayhem, exuded so much dramatic urgency, that he has literally forgotten that there's still a third option: no pet at all.

I act fast, knowing that my time is limited, for Kevin might suddenly realize he's been tricked, and revoke his dog proposal. One week later, having decided not to be allergic anymore, I write a ridiculous, embarrassing $550 check for a puppy with an even more ridiculous, embarrassing namesake: a Westipoo. No, he's not a poor, abused creature from the shelter. There's no higher good associated with this transaction, nothing progressive-minded or benevolent about it. It's just an exchange of goods and services for the pure, selfish, I-don't-give-a-shit purpose of indulging myself in puppy love. Not much different from buying meth on the street, really. We name him Tebow—pronounced TEE-bow—after the Florida Gators football quarterback. Not my idea, but since I got my way with the thing that really mattered—getting a pet in the first place—I figure Kevin should at least be allowed to pick the name.

Besides, our new dog's name is the least of my concerns. What matters most is that I now have this small animal to cart around in a sling, all snug and cozy against my torso. I have him to love, socialize, feed, and train. He's an integral part of my new life.

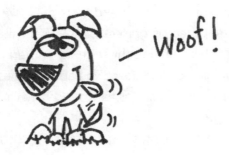

# THE SKY IS BECKONING

KEVIN AND I ARE SITTING AT THE KITCHEN table drinking coffee. He's reading the newspaper, and I'm flipping listlessly through my Betty Crocker cookbook. I come across a glossy, dog-eared page stained with vanilla extract and caked bits of dried dough; it's the cut-out sugar cookie recipe I follow every Christmas, the kind of cookies I would have made in a month or so and frosted with Pillsbury vanilla icing tinted with food coloring. I would have frozen dozens of them in big Zip-Lock bags to bring to Hilton Head and St. Louis for Christmas with our respective families. In that future that isn't going to happen, we would have all sat around and eaten these cookies while passing the new baby from lap to lap.

I close the book and stare out the window at the sunny backyard, which is so overly bright that I practically have to squint. The more I think about it, the less I feel like spending twenty-five hours in airports and airplanes, surrounded by grim fellow travelers and their screaming offspring. Even worse is the thought of being cloistered in a Hilton Head condo with Rob and Mindy and their two babies, babies that aren't mine. My eyes start to water and I blink as hard as I can. Kevin looks up.

"Are you alright?"

I tear off a paper towel, pressing it against my closed eyes for a few seconds, that hot pre-crying sensation passing through my sinuses. My brother's words echo unexpectedly inside of my brain: *Do the things you want to do. Reconnect with who you are.*

"I…yeah. I'm fine. I just…really wish we weren't spending fifteen hundred bucks or whatever just to fly all over hell and creation this Christmas."

"Let's cancel and do something else. What were you thinking?"

I lean against the counter. "I wanna do something that's just...us. The kind of trip we used to do, somewhere overseas. I think we need to reconnect with who we are, like what Paul was saying."

"Arright. Let's plan something."

Gosh, being with Kevin is so easy, it hurts. Within an hour, he's gone online and checked airfares to a bunch of countries. Then, he comes into the bedroom, where I'm reading through the collection of sympathy cards people have sent us over the months, even though I've already read them all ten times.

"How about Ecuador? The flights to Quito aren't bad."

I really don't know anything about Ecuador, but it has a nice ring to it. "Okay."

We cancel our other Christmas tickets without much further thought, and book our two-and-a-half week trip to South America. Afterward, we e-mail our parents, informing them we've decided to do an "our-kind-of-trip" for the holidays. Everyone writes back right away and tells us that sounds like a good idea. Figured they wouldn't argue.

Later that week, Kevin brings home a *Lonely Planet* guide to Ecuador. Scrolling through images of forest-covered mountains and flipping through the "Food" section (always my favorite), I already feel little waves of excitement about our decision, followed by relief about being excited. Because if I couldn't get excited about a trip like this, then I would wonder who on earth I had become.

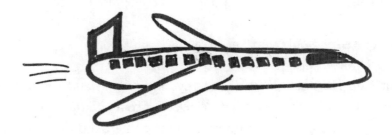

# HOT-TUB MANIA

IT'S A TYPICALLY COLD and rainy evening, and I'm lounging around in my bathrobe and moose slippers, flipping backwards through an issue of *Real Simple* that my mom left for me.  Tebow is curled up on my lap, a little ball of caramel colored fur. Classes are finally going reasonably well, with my students perking up and making me feel like a real teacher, so I'm giving myself the night off from grading as a personal reward. Recently, I've taken to reading magazines backwards so I can soak up all the lighter fluff first. Kevin, predictably, comes through the back door at 10:15.

"Let's jump in the hot tub," he says.

"Hot tub?" I'm utterly confused for a second, for this suggestion seems off-the-wall, not at all a part of our usual bedtime routine. Plus, I've forgotten we even *have* a hot tub, tucked away in a corner of the back yard. When we bought the house, I was pregnant, and hot tubs—of course—are on the list of preggo no-nos. "But...we've never used that thing before. Isn't it all gross?"

"I cleaned it out this morning, so it should be fine. Come on!"

He disappears into the bedroom, and I hear him unzipping his rain jacket.

"It's freezing out there, Kev!" I say.

"Whatever! Let's go!"

It feels like ages since we did anything as wild and spontaneous as jumping in a hot tub past ten o'clock on a cold and rainy weeknight. I get up and go into the bedroom to rummage around for a swimsuit, even though my body is nowhere near the shape it needs to be in for me to wear such a thing. Kevin has already stripped down and has a towel around his waist.

"Wow, that was fast," I say. "Wait, are you, like, *naked* under there?"

"Yup. Hurry up!"

"But I can't find a scrunchie!"

"Who cares! I'll be outside."

This crazy night just got crazier. Not only am I about to jump naked in a hot tub (for I'm certainly not going to be outdone by *Kevin*), but I'm doing it with my hair down. Soaking my already split ends in heavily chlorinated water, which would make most hairdressers cringe. And all of this instigated by Kevin, who doesn't do things like run around naked in the yard! I'm the one in the relationship who's supposed to throw caution to the wind. At least I was, back before I started getting pregnant, since mommies—or pregnant princesses, at least—do only what makes sense for the baby.

I get undressed and slip on my flannel bathrobe over my bare skin, dashing out into the backyard, glancing furtively up toward the neighbors' windows. I doubt anyone's looking, and even if they are, it's their loss for getting a glimpse of my bare, jiggly white arse. Kevin is already sitting in the tub, only his head visible above the glimmering black water. I throw off my robe, my skin instantly tingling and covered with goose bumps from the frigid, drizzly air, and jump in beside him. Sinking down into the hot, swirling water up to my chin, I feel instantly relaxed and melty.

"This is so awesome!" I squeal. "I can't believe we have a hot tub!"

I suppose I've always known it's there, but I just never really saw it. Rising up and floating on my backside, I peer out into the darkness of our yard. Leaves rustle softly and the huge tree in our neighbor's yard forms a jagged silhouette against the purplish nighttime sky. Again, it occurs to me that the neighbors could theoretically see my boobs on the surface of the water if they had binoculars and were really motivated to watch. But Kevin doesn't seem concerned, and he's got a much better sense than I do of what's embarrassing and what's not, so I figure we must be okay. We sit there for a long time and listen to the bubbling water, as I express my amazement every few minutes at the fact that we have this churning cauldron of warmth and happiness right here in our backyard.

"Yup. It's always been here," he says.

For a brief while, about twenty minutes or so, I feel like me again. A whole, undamaged, balanced, non-worrying me. All of this reminds me that I'd better start jogging again and drinking vegetable juice. We ARE going on vacation to someplace presumably sunny, and it would be nice to slip into that dress I wore to the funeral without busting the zipper. And maybe—just maybe—that long lost g-string. If I can find it, that is.

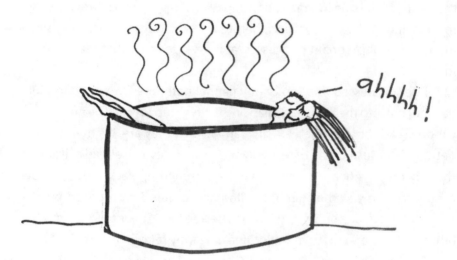

# Going Places

ONLY ONE OF OUR NEIGHBORS KNOWS what happened: Peggy, the sweet, older hippie lady who lives next door with her gay roommate. The only reason I told her is that she popped her head up over the top of the fence while I was sitting on the deck with Tebow, and asked how the baby was doing. I walked over and told her in one sentence what had happened, and her face crumpled. That was that.

But she's the only one. It's not that we're purposely trying to keep it a secret; it's just that we barely know our neighbors, and nobody besides Peggy has inquired. Embarrassingly, Kevin and I have never said more than cursory "hello" to anyone on our block since we moved in five months ago. I hardly want to kick off my effort to be more neighborly by knocking randomly on people's doors and going, "Hi, I'm Monica. Just for the record, the reason I'm not big and round anymore is that I had that baby. Oh, and the baby died, by the way. Great paint job on your front door!"

In my twisted fantasy world, in which everyone is constantly thinking and talking about me, I imagine some nosy old lady gossiping on the phone with the other nosy old lady across the street, both of them watching our house through their living room windows. As I walk down the driveway, Tebow strapped to my torso in his puppy carrier, they try to piece it all together: *clearly she's no longer pregnant, but where's the baby? Did she give birth to a puppy instead? Was she really just fat this whole time? Are they into the baby-trafficking business? Did they sell the baby? Was she a surrogate mother? Did the baby pass away? Surely not that last, horrific one, for she still smiles as she strolls down the driveway, yapping on her cell*

179

*phone. And I know they've had more than one loud, thumping party in that basement of theirs the past few months. That's not something that* people in mourning *do.*

The other, more likely (albeit less thrilling) scenario is that the rest of our block doesn't give a darn about me and my mysterious predicament.

One brisk and cloudy Saturday morning, I discover that at least one neighbor besides Peggy does—in fact—care. After putting on my two sports bras, a long-sleeve t-shirt and my ratty white sneakers, I take two puffs of my inhaler and sprint out onto the sidewalk, breathing in through my nose. Clean morning air, smelling refreshingly of pine needles and cement. Perfect day for a getting-body-ready-for-vacation-mode jog. Just then, Dennis—Peggy's roommate—steps out of his pick-up truck, directly in front of me. He's wearing a black t-shirt that reveals his muscular upper arms. We stop, smile, and say "hey" in unison, and I immediately feel a tad bit of awkwardness over not having made more of a concerted effort to be proactively social with him. He's my next-door neighbor, for God's sake (not to mention hot).

"How's it going?" I say.

His initial smile fades.

"I'm doing fine." He looks directly into my eyes, and I try not to look away. Did I already mention his hotness? "You know, Peggy told me what happened to you guys back in August. I just…God…I know I hardly know you or anything, but it just…makes me so *upset.* You and Kevin are such good, decent people, and it's so terrible that this would happen to you. You didn't deserve something like this…it's not fair!"

His voice quivers and eyes fill up with tears, and I hear him stifle a deep sob. I stand there speechless for a few seconds, surprised and touched by this honest display of sorrow from a person I've never met. Just pure, raw sentiment, the utterly perfect truth: *it's not fair.* But what's bizarre about this conversation—what catches me most off guard—is the way that I feel in contrast: relatively peaceful, steady, my feet on solid ground. He extends his arms toward me and I take that as my cue to give him a long, hard hug, right there on the sidewalk. Hugging a guy I've really only talked to once in my life. His body is hard, the contours of his chest muscles against my face, and I instinctively suck in my stomach. *Thank the lord this man is gay*, I think inwardly, briefly noting that I haven't felt that sort of bodily electric charge in a while. We sniffle into each other's shoulders, and then separate.

I look down at my hands for a minute, wanting suddenly to make Dennis feel better, assure him that this isn't the end of the world, hardly believing my own urge to comfort. Hasn't it been mostly the other way around these past few weeks, months? Years, even?

"Dennis, thanks so much for saying that. It means a lot to me that you can be so honest. It'll be okay. Kevin and I are doing the best we can. Shit happens, ya know?"

He nods and keeps looking at me intensely. "Yeah, shit happens, I guess. Let me know if there's anything that Peggy and I can do. Seriously."

"I will. Thanks, Dennis."

And with that, we both continue on our merry ways. I adjust my sports bra and hair band, and as I cross over the gray freeway, cars roaring beneath my feet, a smile tugs up at the corners of my mouth. Not too long ago, this little exchange would have brought about a meltdown. I would've 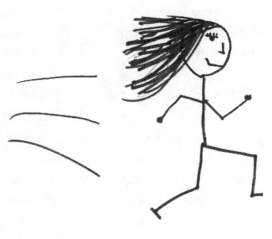 pretended to continue my jog but gone around the block instead, returning to the house and falling into Kevin's arms, my aching heart suddenly aching even more, having soaked up Dennis's sorrow. At least, that's what I think I would have done. I suppose you never know where you are until you look backward, comparing how you felt then to how you feel now.

# TRIBE GATHERING

I'M DRIVING ALONG A NARROW ROAD lined with dense forest. On the radio, nothing. Just silence, the "khshhhh" of frigid, piney air blowing in through the cracked windows of my beat-up Buick sedan. Inside me is the hot, pregnant feeling that something scary and unknown—yet direly meaningful—is about to happen, like when my son's still body was placed into my arms. The road twists suddenly, and I pull on the steering wheel as carefully as a nervous driver can.

Who wouldn't be nervous, driving alone into the woods to spend three days at something called a "Women's Healing Infant-Loss Retreat?" Three days sequestered with total strangers? Just the name itself is cause for suspicion—particularly for non-healing-retreat kinds of people like me. The tiny, under-detailed announcement caught my eye in one of the newsletters that still gets stuffed into our mailbox. I called the organizer, just to make sure it wasn't going to be like Bible camp, or worse—a cult gathering where we all drink poisonous Kool-Aid and commit suicide together. In the forest. Where nobody will find us.

"What is it—like a pow-wow or something?" I said.

Soft chuckle. "No, no. Just a group of six or seven women who went through a recent death of a baby."

"But, like, what'll we be doing for three whole days?"

"Just sharing our stories, doing yoga, getting massages. Lots of time to talk and connect."

Talking and connecting? Getting relaxing rub-downs? Sounded harmless enough, I guess.

Life has been feeling inexplicably lighter lately. Maybe it's from floating naked in the hot tub—which Kevin and I now plunge into almost every night—or the warm, doe-eyed puppy curled up on my lap in the evenings. Whatever it is, I've begun to feel like a helium balloon, floating up and away from earthly, sludge-like thoughts.

Yet something tugged at my insides when I read about the retreat, an urge to drop back down and sink my feet into the damp, brownish earth. Time to return to my tribe—or find them for the first time, actually. And in the words, "Women's Healing Infant-Loss Retreat," I saw the potential way to get there—provided it wasn't Bible camp. So I told Kevin I had to go, and he agreed more quickly than I thought he would.

I turn into a long driveway, finding myself among a cluster of sophisticated cabins and resort-ish buildings backed by more trees and—in the distance—the Olympic Mountains. Who knows how many of the other women are here; could be all six or seven of them, sitting in a circle and chanting in foreign tongues. I push that absurd thought out of my mind and turn off the engine, step into the brisk outdoors, and grab my overstuffed backpack.

As I walk toward the front entrance with gravel crunching beneath my feet, I get a sudden, near-supernatural sense of a presence: Zachary. In the air, reflected in the glass windows and the slate-gray sky above, among the pine trees swaying in the periphery of the parking lot. Not just Zachary, but his little sidekick fetus-brother that came before him. I feel them both swirling around me in tandem, one smaller than the other. Must be all in my head, since ghosts are a bogus concept as far as I'm concerned. Still, goose bumps prick at my forearms as I propel myself forward and open the heavy oak door.

The woman at the front desk sees me, and somehow just knows. "Women's retreat?"

"Yup," I say with eyes downcast. I feel self-conscious, like I'm arriving at a conference for extremely obese or retarded people.

She smiles and comes around to my side, ushering me down a long hallway, and points to a door. "You're the fourth to show up. The others are in here."

I push my way inside. It's a large, carpeted room with leather furniture clustered around a stone fireplace, the gray sky and trees visible through floor-to-ceiling windows. Three normal-looking, pretty women about my age are sitting together on a brown sofa. One of them is clutching a framed picture of an infant hooked up to tubes and machines; I can see it clearly from the doorway. The others are peering at the photo over her hunched shoulders. Brutal awfulness of carrying a baby, delivering, losing: I understand without having to ask. I close the door behind me, and the three women look up in unison.

"Monica?"

"Yeah."

"I'm Carla, the organizer. We talked on the phone. I'm so glad you made it. This is Lindsey and Vicky."

They all stand up and I drop my bag to the floor, the self-consciousness of twenty seconds ago evaporating through my shoulders. This isn't Jesus camp or a poisonous Kool-Aid cult after all! And this isn't Marge and Candace from the Fayetteville support group either, staring down at me with disapproving eyes. Without thinking, I stride toward the group and collapse against each woman in a hard, prolonged hug; no need for hellos here. I feel oddly buoyed, comforted—as though I've stumbled into a homecoming gathering with kindred friends who have been here all along, traveling with me down this lonesome, half-mom-half-not path. It just took a while to find them. We all sink into the leather sofa, nestling together.

"They gave him to us so we could wait for him to die," says Lindsey, straw-colored hair pulled back off her stunningly pretty face as she peers at that photo of the baby attached to tubes. "It took eleven hours."

*Wait for him to die.*

Could've been Zachary, could've been me. I rest one hand on her forearm and tilt my head back on the cushion behind me, breathing in deeply.

*This is our tribe, Zachary. We finally found 'em.*

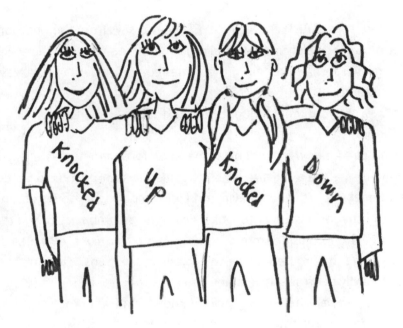

# Return of the G-String

"HAVE YOU STARTED PACKING YET?" Kevin says from the bedroom as I sit on the edge of the bathtub, clipping my toenails into the toilet, enjoying the satisfying sound of the blades coming together. "We leave in forty minutes."

"Crap. Are you sure? I thought we had...like...at least an hour."

"Nope."

I'm not sure how it suddenly came to be forty minutes—well, now thirty-nine—before a shuttle bus is scheduled to transport us to Seatac International Airport, where Kevin and I will embark on a series of long flights to Ecuador, a country to which I've given an embarrassingly little amount of thought aside from a quick glance at our *Lonely Planet*. Life has been so firmly rooted in the weirdness and responsibilities of here that I've hardly been able to imagine being elsewhere, let alone a foreign country. It's a Spanish-speaking place, I know. Somewhat mountainous. Possibly sidles up against an ocean, but can't remember for sure. The only trip planning I've really done is driven Tebow to the home of a nice, young lady that dog-sits for twenty-five bucks a day. I found her in the classifieds, and told her to take good care of my little baby-substitute. She gave a strange look and laughed nervously when I said it.

A frantic flurry of activity ensues as I drag my dusty old backpack out of the basement closet, racing around the house and stuffing it with anything that seems more or less suitable for a vacation. A bar of soap and a new razor. A can of vegetable juice for the plane. A red spiral notebook for recording deep thoughts, of which I am bound to have many while I'm sitting on the beach. If there is a beach.

I yank the huge cardboard box labeled "summer clothes" out of the closet, and empty it onto the floor. Brightly colored tank tops, sun dresses, form-fitting t-shirts spill out, all wrinkled and still streaked with white deodorant marks from having not been washed in over a year. Oh well, too late now. After hurriedly picking out a few favorites, I throw the rest back into the box, and then pull open my top dresser drawer to grab a fistful of faded Hanes briefs.

Just as I'm about to slam the drawer shut, I notice a flash of pink, way in the back behind the socks and wire cup bras. It takes me a few seconds to recognize it. *G-string panties. Christmas 2005.* Two years ago. An ancient-seeming artifact, neglected and forgotten, from that distant era when my body was more than just a perpetually-ten-pounds-overweight holding cell for hope, grief, more hope, and more grief. Frankly, I'm shocked this neglected article of clothing made it all the way from Arkansas.

As a horn honks loudly in the driveway, I impulsively grab the wadded-up g-string and cram it into my backpack alongside everything else. My body is hardly a temple of passion these days, but what the hell. This is a *vacation* after all, which used to mean a time to let loose, break free of the granny underwear identity, slurp down sugary cocktails and do sensual things in bed. I also snag my dark blue one-piece swimsuit from the hall closet too. Again, just in case there's a beach.

There is a beach, it turns out. I only know this because twenty-four hours of traveling later, a beat up taxi drops us off on a dusty road at Punta Ayampe, a smattering of wooden cabanas perched on a lush hillside overlooking the Pacific Ocean. We are ushered to our open-air cabin, permanently gritty with windblown sand and creaking on its four posts, with no electricity or human sounds—just the distant roar of crashing waves. With the exception of the proprietor, a skinny long-haired man, Kevin and I have the entire place to ourselves. After throwing down our backpacks, we plop down on the edge of the bed and look at each other.

"Well, here we are," says Kevin. He pulls a pair of green swim trunks out of his bag. "I'm gonna go see if they have a surfboard I can use."

"Okay. How long are we planning on staying here?" I don't know why I feel the need to know that.

"Who knows. However long we feel like. I told them two nights but that's not etched in stone."

"Mmm-kay," I say, feeling a twinge of worry that two nights might be too long in a place this quiet, this free of people and activities and tasks to distract me from inadvertently brooding. Fear that I might not remember how to do nothing, or that I might start seriously missing my dog. Or Zachary. There isn't even Internet service out here.

"I'm gonna take a quick shower," I say. "I'll meet you at the beach."

Peeling off my jeans and t-shirt and sweaty wire-cup bra, I grab the razor and oatmeal soap that I brought from home, and step into our white tiled shower. The water is cool and clear and earthy smelling; I can see that it comes from a plastic tank outside. There's a large, high window in the shower wall, looking out over tropical foliage; any old bird or lizard could probably see me naked in here. But that doesn't bother me.

As I scrape the razor along my calves, armpits, and bikini line, tapping the blades against the wall to clean them of clumps of dark body hair, I realize I haven't shaved since the funeral. Lovely, Monica. I can clearly envision the look of disdain that would cross Kevin's face if he were to see me doing this in our own shower (I know he knows that I do this regularly).

Then, I get out and run my fingers through my wet hair, rub Burt's Bees lotion all over my skin, and dig up a crumpled, somewhat formfitting cotton dress and a pair of clean underwear (the nice, safe granny ones, of course, which cover my entire butt with wholesome flowers and rise up to the bottom of my ribcage).

Already I'm starting to feel physically better and lighter, now stripped free of body hair and those heavy, airplane-smelling clothes. I walk out onto the creaking balcony, looking out at the shimmering blue strip of ocean between the treetops. Breathing in deep through my nose, I am keenly aware that this is one of the earth's beautiful and perfect places, and I try to concentrate for a minute on appreciating it, being fully present, enjoying the distant pulsating roar of the ocean waves.

*Vacation mode, Monica. Not worrying-about-nothing mode. Remember how to do this?*

Swallowing hard, I go back inside and pull off my granny-undies, slipping on that g-string instead. It's the first time I've worn it in nearly two years.

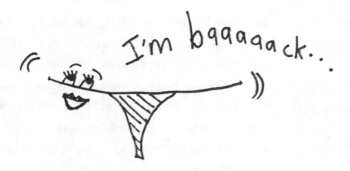

KEVIN AND I QUICKLY SLIP into a bare bones routine of sleeping in late, eating lots of seafood cooked in butter and garlic, walking barefoot in the sand, wading out into the ocean and bobbing up and down, and—yes—screwing. The g-string doesn't go unnoticed, with Kevin running his fingers and mouth along the edge of them.

"I like you in these," he says. "Your skin tastes salty."

I feel tingly all over, which I haven't felt in forever. Just a few traces of it when Dennis hugged me on the sidewalk, but that's about it. As one day melts into two and three, I still think of Zachary in my belly, of the Christmas we would have spent with our families in my former future, but without so much desperate pining as before.

It isn't until a full week later that we decide it's time to move on to the mountainous interior on a ramshackle, smoke-spewing bus. Here, while wandering through a little village ringed with towering green peaks—we discover a wooden sign hanging on a whitewashed door: *Overnight Horse Treks Here.*

Instantly, my heart does a little flip, because this is something I would have gotten excited about long ago, before the prospect of baby-making began trumping all other excitements. I crave trying it—right now—although I know that bouncing around on horseback isn't Kevin's type of thing. And the idea of going off without him, of doing something completely by myself (let alone in a foreign country), is more unnerving than I care to admit. Still, if being alive means doing the things you love, then I simply have to do this—even if it means going solo.

So I swallow down that fear of aloneness, deftly keeping it a secret from Kevin, and we French-kiss and part ways for several days with a plan to meet back in Quito. He goes off to join a cycling excursion, while I head up into the wilderness on the back of a large beast with a ruddy-faced guide and a handful of other tourists. We ascend up into the mountains; pure blue sky, rocky cliffs, and a green valley below with a sparkling stream snaking along the bottom of it. I breathe in through my nose, sitting up tall and patting the sweaty skin under my horse's mane, gazing down at the marvelous scenery around me.

For two nights, we stay at a tin-roofed hut overlooking the valley. Our guide cooks some kind of meaty stew over an open fire, and we all clamor into his little fire-lit cooking area and eat together, scraping our plates loudly with our forks and laughing. Toward the end of the meal, he produces a bottle of cheap vodka and five mugs, pouring each of us a hefty serving. This must be his signature welcome gift. We clink glasses and down our drinks, conversing into the wee hours of the night about typical things that travelers discuss when they encounter one another: where we're from, where we've traveled before, where we're headed. Just normal topics that I used to talk about.

I can't wait to tell Kevin about it, about the scent and sight of this remote corner of the earth, about the conversations, about the fact that I rode for seven hours in my g-string (which has been washed several times in saltwater and is now wedged halfway up my arse). Come to think of it, it's been a while since there was anything that I couldn't wait to tell Kevin about. My gut tells me this is a good sign.

## Spinning Sex Machine

WANDERING AIMLESSLY THROUGH Quito's narrow streets, dodging buses puffing black smoke, I pause to look upward at fragments of blue sky between the tops of Spanish colonial buildings. Calm, electrifying blue above the city. I stumble across a grassy expanse, a large city park dotted with fountains and swing sets, stopping to buy a hunk of cold watermelon from a dark skinned woman in a pink dress. She's got an infant swaddled up against her chest, which makes my stomach do a barely perceptible flip. I wonder with mild irritation if that little baby-induced flip will ever stop happening. I say "Gracias" and find a shady spot, where I sit down Indian-style and lick the sweet watermelon juice now running down my wrists.

This will be my second night in this sprawling, foreign city by myself. Kevin will be here tonight, thank goodness. The solitude is good and all, but starts to get old after a while. I feel like a paper doll in this urban sea of people, unknown and anonymous, practically invisible. No television in our homey, orange-and-yellow painted guesthouse, which means no Ecuadorian newscasters and suit-clad game show hosts keeping me company in incomprehensible Spanish. No possible way to reach Kevin, since I don't even know the name of the mountain-bike tour company that he's with—although I suppose if I started acting hysterical, the smiling young woman at the front desk would help me track him down with the help of the city police.

I finish my watermelon, gnawing away at the rind until I reach the hard bitter part, and start walking back toward our hotel for a nap. Just as

I'm about to turn onto our street, I notice a handwritten paper sign taped to the weathered front door of an old building. It says:

*"Salsa Lessons $5! We Are Open!"*

I stop in the middle of the sidewalk, staring at the sign. This is the second intriguing sign of the trip, the first being that of overnight horse trek, both presenting some form of seemingly cosmic opportunity. If I really believed in an otherworldly being controlling the gears up there, I would think that he—or she—must be leading me to these signs so they can serve some mysterious greater purpose in my life.

I push on the door and it creaks open slowly, revealing a dark and shadowy stairwell. Above is the muffled sound of thumping music, exuberant and rhythmic, beckoning me to come up. Salsa lessons are something that Kevin would reluctantly do, but only to make me happy, and only if sufficiently intoxicated and cajoled. After feeling around in my back pocket and making sure that some cash is there, I decide to take this one on—and up the dark and shadowy stairwell I go. At the top, a door opens to a bright and sunny office, where I am greeted by a smiling woman with the perfect body of a dancer.

"Lesson?" she asks.

"*Sí*," I tell her.

"One hour, five dollars. *¿Bueno?*"

Considering that a salsa lesson at the dance studio next to Green Lake costs fourteen or twenty times that much (I've checked), I'd say yeah, that's "*bueno.*" So I hand her a crumpled bill. Without asking what my experience level is, which I'd say is "beginner plus" since I do have quite a few dance parties under my belt, she takes my hand and pulls me down a narrow hallway. There are group lessons going on around us—I can see glimpses of them through various doorways, mostly older white people dancing in pairs as native instructors call out steps in broken English. I fully expect to be led into one of these groups, because for a mere five dollars, I'm certainly not going to insist on a one-on-one tutorial. But we pass all of these doorways, and instead she guides me into a spacious room with hardwood floors and a full wall of mirrors, empty except for a CD player with enormous speakers in the corner. Sunlight pours in through the large windows looking out over the busy street.

"One minute. Teacher come," she says, and then disappears in a cloud of perfume, closing the door behind her.

Standing in the middle of the quiet room alone, I don't quite know what to do with myself. I examine my head-to-toe reflection in the mirror, adjusting my hair barrettes. A formfitting, navy blue t-shirt, ratty white sneakers, slightly hip-hugging jeans with granny Hanes briefs hidden underneath them. I discovered on the horse trek that wearing a g-string isn't so fun when there isn't anyone to wear it for.

I wonder what other people see when they look at me. I've always been told I have a "generically ethnic look," with my dark eyebrows and hair. Am I young? Seductive? Ish? I had just begun to feel this way at Punta Ayampe, a feeling I thought had been buried forever. Turning sideways, I suck in my stomach and stick my chest out just a tad, extending my arms to embrace an invisible partner, swaying back and forth on the balls of my feet. I can almost imagine myself on stage with a—

*"Hola."*

Startled, I breathe in sharply and release my stomach from its sucked-in position, spinning around toward the mysterious voice. Leaning against the doorframe is a man with about the finest body I've ever seen in person, watching me. A shadow obscures his face, but I can clearly depict his well-defined arm muscles and caramel-color skin. Some combination of black and Hispanic, probably in his early twenties, maybe even nineteen. He's wearing a white tank top stretched tight across his built upper body, and black jogging pants that rest low and perfect on his hips. His whole appearance—the way he leans with his head tilted just so, the way his clothes hang lazily on his body causes my heart rate to shoot up. I say a quick prayer that he's not the teacher, for that would be just too much to process.

*"Hola,"* I say nervously. "Um, lesson?"

He shuts the door behind him and saunters toward me, the corners of his mouth still turned up in a handsome half-grin. As he comes into the light, I can see that his face is just as mind-bogglingly beautiful as his body, his mouth and jaw perfect, nose straight, teeth white. We shake hands and he introduces himself as something like "Xavier," and then says a string of things in Spanish, his voice low and quiet.

"*No comprendo,*" I say, agonizingly self-conscious.

"*No problemo.*"

He walks to the CD player in the corner and presses play.

*But there is a "problemo,"* I think to myself as music, loud and whimsical, fills the room. *You are too damned young and hot for a beginner salsa teacher, and there is no way I'm going to learn anything with your hands on my body.*

He returns to my side, looking straight at me, pointing first to his eyes and then to his feet. I watch and concentrate. He steps and counts. *Uno, dos, tres.* I imitate his footwork, imagining that I'm with a nice, safe, comfy group of elderly white people at a retirement home instead of in a room alone with this impossibly hunky man. It's the only way I can keep my knees from turning to gelatin. We both face the mirror and do it together, repeating the pattern that he showed me, my eyes trained on his feet. He doesn't tell me "good" or anything; in fact, he says nothing at all, thoughtfully watching my steps and my face, nodding periodically. I find myself wanting to impress him, and relieved whenever I see him nod, which I interpret as a sign of approval.

Then, without warning, he slips his arm around my waist and pulls me toward him effortlessly, guiding my arms and hands into place. The top of my head almost reaches his chin, and if I look up, I come face-to-face with his achingly distracting mouth. So I look down at my feet instead, biting my lower lip, a tense feeling inside my chest. He puts fingers beneath my chin and pulls my head up, pointing to my eyes and then to his. Compelling me to hold his gaze, which I can only do for about three seconds before coming undone and staring at the floor again.

We dance like this for some time, turning and moving across the room as I awkwardly follow his smooth and confident lead. Every few minutes we stop, and he shows me another pattern, and then we resume dancing together, blending new steps with old ones. Whenever I take my eyes off his, he catches it instantly like the "eye contact KGB," pulling my chin up, holding his hand there for several seconds and looking intently into my eyes. Demanding that I do it right. I personally think he should be cutting me some slack, considering what I've been through this past year-and-a-half—although I don't blame him for not knowing my history.

Just as we start getting into what I consider a decent groove, he abruptly stops, pushing back from me with both hands. I stand there panting, aware of the sheen of sweat that has formed on my lower back, and watch him quizzically. Is it already break time? Or is he tired of me, frustrated that I can't maintain eye contact? With a dead serious expression, he points to my hips and then to his, which he starts to sway seductively, like a snake. Realizing what he's trying to teach me, I swallow hard, attempting to mimic his fluid hip motions. Honestly, I want to tell him, it's okay if I don't master the perfect "Latino sway" this go around; just picking up a few steps is good enough for me. But clearly, it isn't good enough for him.

Closing in so that he's standing a mere half-inch away, so unnervingly near that I can smell faint whispers of salt and cologne on his young skin, he lifts my hands up and plants them around his neck. *This must be some modern Ecuadorian high school-dance version of salsa,* I think to myself. Then he runs his fingertips slowly down the slopes of my bare arms, over my shoulders and along the length of my torso to my hips, leaving a trail of tingly numbness the whole way. A warm sensation starts in my core, spreading throughout my limbs. Gently, he moves my hips from side to side, right in sync with his.

With my face almost squarely against his chest, his warm breath at my forehead, I sense him commanding me to do the impossible: to shed the tired construct of myself as a Hanes-wearing gringo, a beginner student, a mere dead baby factory, and see myself as something more. To stop trying so hard to get the damn footwork right, and trust myself to move naturally like a real dancer, sexy and uninhibited. To let myself go.

*If only you knew how much you're asking of me.* If he realized how faraway I am from ever being a real dance starlet, if he understood that I

195

recently delivered a six-pound dead baby, if he knew how often I still wake up with the post-crying face of a puffer fish, if he sensed my reproductive and motherly inferiority, if he saw that I was wearing granny-undies beneath these arse-hugging jeans, he would never hold me to such high expectations. He would feel sorry for me, tolerating my stiff and mechanical posture and glancing at the clock, eager for his time dancing with a piece of prudish plywood to be over.

But he can't know those things, and I don't have the Spanish to tell him, which means they can't be legitimately used as excuses for being a shitty amateur. Still yearning to please him, I finally allow my hips to move the way they should, tugged along by the music and Xavier's strong hands. He pulls back and we return to a civilized and traditional salsa pose, except that this time I feel more confident and relaxed than before. The tenseness has evaporated from my torso, for no reason other than a conscious shift in the way I see myself, and I lock my eyes on Xavier's for the first time, unafraid. His expression remains serious, but his eyes seem to now have a new, subtle sparkle. Or perhaps I'm just imagining it. We dance like this for song after song, our allotted time spilling over what I've paid for—at least according to the clock on the windowsill—until Xavier finally stops and looks at me, pointing to his eyes.

By now, I know this means it's my turn to wait with anticipation and watch, for he's going to teach me what is probably the final new move of the day. We're both breathing hard and damp with sweat, and I brush a thick strand of hair out of my face. Unexpectedly, he slips his hand behind my knee, lifts up my leg, and wraps it around him, standing so that my other foot is planted between his.

I become hyper aware of his crotch pressed against me, and—I would swear on the Holy Bible if asked—it feels…*almost feels*…like he has a hard-on. Literally, like there's a rock behind his fly. I can't imagine that could possibly be, for that would be so sinfully inappropriate that I might just die right here and now. So I imagine it as a sock ball instead. Before I know what's happening, he braces my lower back with his hand and dips me so far backward that I instinctively resist. As I struggle to stand back upright, he shakes his head and says something in Spanish.

*Relax, I'll hold you,* I feel him saying. Or perhaps he's saying, *You're making my penis hard.*

I wonder.

I take a deep breath and nod, pinning him against me once more with my leg, briefly acknowledging again the close proximity of his cement-like, 3-D crotch, and allow myself to free fall as though I'm doing a back bend. This time, I dip so low that the top of my head almost touches the floor behind me, trusting Xavier's strong arm to keep me from cracking my noggin open. He pulls me swiftly back up, my head spinning and cheeks flushed, and we continue dancing like this until the song ends, finishing with one more perfect backward dip.

The last song on the CD finishes with impeccable timing, the room now totally silent. Xavier and I remain pressed against each other for a few frozen seconds as I unwrap my leg from the backs of his thighs. His head is bent down toward mine, his breath warm, and his hands slide down my backside, lingering there for a moment. And then he steps back.

"*Gracias,*" he says, smiling that half-smile again, and turns to walk out. And with that, he's gone.

I stare after him speechlessly, disbelievingly, crestfallen, my throat dry, trying to fathom how our five-dollar hour could already be over. I was just starting to get that backward dip, just getting used to the idea of myself as this newly confident, hip-swaying person who looks my hot-ass partner bravely in the eye and—quite possibly, although I'll never know for sure—gives him an erection. Still panting and somewhat dazed, I wander out into the main office.

"Um, *yo quiero* another salsa lesson," I say to the smiling woman with the dancer's body, holding out my second five-dollar bill of the afternoon.

"Five minutes we close," she says.

"*¿Mañana?*" I say, but she shakes her head.

"*Mañana* we close."

And since we're leaving on Monday morning, that's it—no more salsa lessons. No more Xavier. Feeling empty and lightheaded, I make my way back down the shadowy stairwell and out into the street, my body still sweaty and feeling oversexed, my skin vibrating. Everything around me seems surreal, cartoonish, as though I just got snatched up and sent through some kind of sex machine, shot into an alternate universe filled with beautiful people and music, reshaped into a lithe and sensual dance star, and then spit back out onto a noisy Quito sidewalk.

Still reeling, I take a circuitous route back to our hotel, searching frantically for other "Salsa Lessons!" signs. If I can find a different place that's open tomorrow, I can sign up for four or five lessons in a row, returning to that strange and sexy salsa universe. I have enough money in my back pocket, and I don't mind paying in advance. But I only find one place, and when I peer in the window, I see that the teacher is a bone thin, long-haired, fair-skinned man of average looks. Certainly not a Xavier, not the mysterious and authoritative type that would inspire me to sway my hips. And besides, they're closed on Sundays too.

So I return to my hotel room and take a long, hot shower. I feel strangely rejuvenated, reinvented, wistfully longing for more of that world of which I got a single sweet taste, hardly enough to satisfy in the long term. Without a second thought, I put on my g-string undies and one of Kevin's t-shirts, which somehow wound up in my backpack, and throw myself on the bed. I can tell this shirt has gone a week or longer without being washed, because it's got the familiar scent of his sweat and Speedstick deodorant concentrated in the armpits, which—although Kevin will never claim to understand—is one of my favorite fragrance combinations on earth. My mind ticks away as I stare up at the ceiling and reflect on today's dreamlike events. Glimpses of myself in the mirror with Xavier, layers of fear stripped away, music thumping and soul-filling. Me, a real living dancer. A hard-on giver.

Kevin shows up late that night, unshaven and slightly sunburned. His cutest and sexiest look, in my opinion. He finds me lounging on an orange overstuffed sofa in the corner of our room with my bare legs slung over the side of it, a closed book on my chest, tears streaming down my face.

"Hey. What's—"

"C'mere—I'm fine." I sniffle and sit up, siding over to make room as I wipe my eyes with my forearm. "Just opened some random book from the shelf and read the middle chapter. It's about a woman's dog getting hit by a car. I missed you. How was the biking?"

We sit and hold hands with my legs draped over his, talking for hours about the details of our separate journeys. I tell him about the bumpy horse trek, the watermelon in the park, the salsa lesson with Xavier, the way I looked in the mirror with his arms around me, even the way his body looked. I leave out the part about the alleged hard-on, though. No point in bringing up something for which I only have circumstantial evidence.

That night, Kevin and I have the best sex I can remember in a very, very long time. Aliveness: check.

# APPENDIX

## HIGHLY UNSCIENTIFIC, POST-TRIP FIELD NOTES FOR THE NEWLY KNOCKED-DOWN

1. CONGRATULATIONS: you just got royally screwed! Something very bad happened to you through no fault of your own, and you are now one of *those people* that bad things happen to, the people you hear about on local news. This particular calamity has been successfully avoided by millions of other individuals (people far less smart and well-intentioned than you, no doubt), as evidenced by the earth's ongoing population explosion. Which means that you should feel special, getting singled out by Mother Nature like this.

2. Actually, forget I said that. Your situation is not unique. 4.5 million stillbirths occur worldwide each year*, with an even greater number of miscarriages. I hate to tell you this, but there are probably more Knocked-Downers in your vicinity than you ever realized, and if you could call them out of the woodwork with a special whistle or code word, they would appear in droves. (Just don't expect them to all come running unprovoked, though. For reasons I have yet to figure out, Knocked Down-ness isn't one of those circumstances that most survivors wear proudly on their sleeves, like alcoholism or breast cancer—although perhaps one of us could design a special black t-shirt or a ribbon we all wear to highlight our status as Dead-Baby-Mommas-n-Daddas. That way we could easily

find each other.) The point is that your invisible Knocked- Down Badge of Honor is not as special as you might sadistically hope.

3.  Actually, never mind. You are special. So is the baby or fetus that slipped away from you—and I don't mean that in a condescending, first-grade-self-esteem-building kind of way. Not to state the obvious, but when you and your spooge-daddy (or spooge-vacuum) got together, your unique sets of genes formed an unprecedented new entity. No other living entity on earth was created with that particular gene combination. An important, irreplaceable piece of you vanished once this small being— or clump of cells or however you choose to think about it—passed away. You may even be able to imagine with hurtful clarity the parent you would have been, the bright future that would have unfolded, the unique child and eventual adult that this particular being would have become. That's why this baby or fetus or pre-fetus—and all of the intangible elements swirling around him or her—deserve to be mourned just like any other death.

4.  But here's what sucks. Other people's trauma is beyond the conversational comfort zone of most people, particularly when it involves the loss of an entity that never had a public face. Most of the world (yourself included) might not view your circumstance as a death at all, but as something else—some vaguely sad and disappointing occurrence without a clear definition—particularly if your pregnancy ended in its very early stages. This can make it difficult to know how or what to mourn, and equally challenging for your friends and family members to know what to say around you. In fact, you might be astounded by the human ability to avoid discussing unpleasant subjects—even big, glaringly obvious shit-storms such as your own loss—as though they never occurred in the first place. This can be especially problematic during the holiday season, when somebody is missing from the family table, and you sense that missing person more acutely than everyone else. It can be a lonely and frustrating experience, to say the least.

5.  But here's what doesn't suck. Most people in your life—with a few exceptions, of course—are fully aware of that missing person at

the table, and saddened in their own way. Although they might not feel comfortable mentioning it, your loss is theirs too. Baby-death is a blow to the entire community. There just aren't any clear-cut rules for how to talk about it.

6. In a land without rules, thou shalt fend for thyself. Did I mention that you just got royally screwed? As in, ravaged on the inside? You're in survival mode right now. This means that you can—*and should, damn it!*—do whatever in heck's name you feel like doing when it comes to avoiding potentially dicey events, like holidays and baby showers (as long as it doesn't involve breaking the law, of course. Legend has it that prisons aren't very conducive to grieving). Skip what you feel like skipping, confer with your partner if you have one, and come up with a plan to do something totally self-pampering. Never mind the rules and traditions, or what others think is best for you, or what your family wants. People will deal with whatever you decide to do. A spa retreat, perhaps? A weekend getaway to a cabin in the woods? A movie-marathon night preceded by ice cream for dinner? Or maybe a Pants-Off-Dance-Off in your basement with friends and blaring rock-n-roll music? Make them all remove their lower garments and hang them at the front door before entering, no exceptions. Or, if family is what you need, demand some quality mom-n-dad time. Follow your gut instinct here.

7. Speaking of survival, have you noticed the amazing survival-tools already built into your body and brain? Here's a perfect example: in the first few hours and days after the Knock Down, your brain will likely be coated in a pleasantly awful film of numbness. Enjoy it while it lasts! One important benefit of this post-trauma high is that it enables you engage in coherent conversation with your doctor. This is important, because your doctor is going to give you all kinds of fun instructions for caring for your knocked down body—things like applying cooling gelatin to your bruised private parts, or sitting on the toilet and waiting for "the thing" to pass. You'll appreciate this list of tangible tasks for bettering your physical state, and the semblance of control it provides—especially now that you have unwillingly learned how little control you really have over

your reproductive destiny. There's also your body's ability to cry, which—when done at the right moment—can be almost as satisfying as a good session of puking or having sex. When nothing else seems to help, these cheap bodily thrills can make all the difference.

8.  I hate to break it to you, but…not only is your forced journey into Knocked-Downville just beginning, but it never really ends. It's not as though five months go by, you press your crotch up against a sexy Latino man's pelvis, and boom—everything is back to normal. Nope: you've been changed in ways that may not be apparent to you now. You know things that you didn't before, and this will likely color your views, actions, and any other future pregnancy that you have. You'll have lots of downs and ups, and then the ups will become more frequent. The downs will never disappear forever, though. That's what trauma does to a person: hits us, hurts us, teaches us, transforms us. I know that sounds totally corny and self-helpish, but it's true.

9.  A final dose of Pollyanna: You might not want to hear something as seemingly dismissive of your pain as what I'm about to say. If fact, it could very well cause you to throw this book out the window or use it as kindling for your next bonfire. But given what you've survived so far, I'm fairly certain you can handle these words too: *although your journey will never end, things ultimately get better*. There, I said it. Have faith in yourself to uncover coping mechanisms you never knew you had, to find your own ways to balance grieving with healing. News flash: they happen at the same time, without you even knowing it. So even as you sit at the holiday dinner table feeling like a big ball of shit, that shit-feeling is part of your healing journey. Aside from your own powerful psyche and soul, the simple passage of time is another one of nature's greatest healers. If you happen to be a Newly Knocked-Downer, you haven't much time under your belt to soothe the rawness and help scar tissue form. But as time goes by, your loss will get folded deeper inside of you, and next year's holidays will be easier than this year's.

I WRITE THIS FROM MY SUNNY LIVING ROOM, exactly two years and six months after Zachary's death. Since then I've had another miscarriage (what is UP with that?), stocked up on more g-string undies (hell, I couldn't keep wearing that one sweaty pair forever), drunk a lot of white Zinfandel, studied Zachary's photos, put them away, dug them back up, biked through Eastern Europe and Ireland with that hot-bodied man of mine, had lots of sex, become a daytime coffee addict, and alternately cried and laughed a whole bunch. The Baby Ladies have, remarkably, remained steadfastly in my life as loyal friends, and I'm finally learning how to see their children as awesome miracles instead of searing reminders of what could have been. I've kept in touch with the gals from the infant loss retreat, too. Most of them have since had subsequent babies, and I'm happy for them. Zachary's death has brought my and Kevin's nomadic families together; it didn't take long for my parents to pack up and move across the country to be closer to us, and Kevin's parents now visit more often than ever before.

At this moment, I'm eight months pregnant with yet another boy. And on the off-chance that this boy turns into a bona fide child—which I finally understand is never a guarantee—I already know what Kevin and I will tell ourselves (and maybe even him) when life deals him hardships: things will get better.

*That's according to the International Stillbirth Alliance. Come on; you think I would pull a number like that out of my arse?

## Acknowledgements

Tremendous thanks go out to my amazing family and friends, whose constant support gave me the courage to persevere wtih this project.

To Kristen Degan, best Peace Corps buddy and personal cheerleader from the moment I started puting my thoughts into words.

To Mom, Dad, and Paul, for helping me see myself as a real writer.

To Jessica Powers of Catalyst Book Press for believing in me.

To N, C, and J—my Seattle Baby-Lady friends—whose relentless friendship, generosity, and compassion have shown what it means to be human.

To knocked-down mommies everywhere, for the strength and inspiration you provide.

To Zachary and Male Fetus, who I hope are witnessing all of this from the MTV Penthouse for Bitchin' Stillborn Babes above.

Most of all, to Kevin LeMoine, my best friend and truest love on earth. He has been the quiet driving force behind this book since the very beginning, and without him it would surely have become a deleted file on a dusty laptop. Kevin, I love you.